"These wide-ranging and thoughtful essays address a theme most vital in our time, the problem of how people move from the grievance response to collective injuries and their unhealed wounds into the mourning process that attenuates further harm. This excellent volume will be most useful and stimulating reading for all who are interested in widening the social scope of psychoanalysis and deepening its involvement with the reactions to traumatic history."

Jessica Benjamin, *PhD author of* Beyond Doer and Done To: Recognition Theory, Intersubjectivity and the Third, *Routledge 2018*

"As contemporary psychoanalysts of all persuasions grapple with the role of the social with regard to both its clinical considerations and its implications for theory, this important and timely book rises to the challenge. This volume comprises a select collection of thoughtful psychoanalytic authors who address questions not of whether the social is part of psychoanalysis but, rather, how the domains of the social and the contextual may be thoughtfully, richly, and fruitfully engaged. Filled with gems of psychoanalytic engagement with social systems, this volume represents a potent response to calls from both within psychoanalysis for theoretical expansion and from a wider world in distress, to which psychoanalytic thinkers are uniquely poised to contribute."

Anton Hart, *PhD, FABP, FIPA*

"A provocative invitation. Dobrich, in an all-hands-on deck approach, provides a multidisciplinary challenge to traditional ways of understanding power, community, and change in our current moment of political crisis. How can practitioners facilitate individuals' understanding of themselves through their community (un)belonging? How do our concepts of self, reflect our group memberships and our individual or group relationships to out-groups? This volume offers a variety of contexts to explore these questions, inviting us to let down our guard and explore who we could be – if we risked curiosity."

Anna Mahoney, *Ph.D., executive director and senior policy fellow, Dartmouth College*

"*Moving from Grievance to Hope in Psychoanalysis: Applied Case Studies*, edited by Johanna Dobrich, offers a timely and compelling vision of applied contemporary psychoanalysis as an ethically engaged, socially responsive praxis. Through illuminating essays by psychoanalytic clinical educators and others, the volume expands the psychoanalytic field beyond the consulting room to address fractured socio-political realities—trauma, extremism, racism, displacement, erasure, and collective grief—while maintaining rigorous attention to relational process. These richly textured case studies trace a developmental movement from inchoate exchanges toward mature intersubjectivity, where self and other are held in mutual recognition, shared meaning, and collective witnessing. Dobrich advances a dynamic, co-constructed psychoanalytic matrix that integrates internal and external worlds, enabling movement from binary, paranoid–schizoid positions toward integrative communal minds without sacrificing individual identity. This compellingly readable collection offers a vital new ethic of responsibility and care in psychoanalytic work and has my strongest endorsement."

Maurice Apprey, *PhD, DM, FIPA, professor emeritus of Psychiatry and Neurobehavioral Sciences, University of Virginia School of Medicine*

"Contemporary psychoanalytic theory and psychoanalytic communities are in crisis, shaped by multiple, and at times mutually inflicted, historical traumas. Yet psychoanalysis has always evolved through engagement with novel social and political challenges, particularly in its understanding of trauma and social trauma. Each theoretical revision has sought to correct earlier exclusions, invalidations, or dismissals of traumatic realities. From Freud's reinterpretation of sexual abuse as fantasy to the misattribution of Holocaust trauma, and later, Vietnam veterans' suffering, as constitutional vulnerability, psychoanalysis has repeatedly struggled to recognize how massive trauma can undo established psychic defenses. In a contemporary climate where sociopolitical ideologies threaten to flatten psychoanalytic depth, this book offers a vital intervention, affirming the coexistence of multiple trauma legacies within a complex global landscape and within psychoanalytic communities themselves. The plurality of perspectives gathered here underscores psychoanalysis's ethical responsibility to foster integration amid psychic and social fragmentation."

Irit Felsen, *PhD, clinical psychologist, adjunct professor of Psychology at Columbia University, and internationally published expert on trauma and intergenerational transmission*

"Dobrich's timely volume brings together an array of brilliant psychoanalytic thinkers to address with rich clinical illustrations and powerful theory the subject of intergenerational trauma. Viewed through family, community, and collective lenses, this volume is a must-read for clinicians and interested laypeople alike."

Grant H. Brenner, *MD, DFAPA, co-chair, Disaster, Trauma and Global Health Committee, Group for the Advancement of Psychiatry*

Moving from Grievance to Hope in Psychoanalysis

This volume brings psychoanalytic thinking and practice directly into the social forces that shape our lives, covering intergenerational trauma, cultural difference, divisive ideologies, environmental degradation, and entrenched social hierarchies.

Through clinical case studies from leading thinkers in the field, the contributors each show how analysts work in social and collective spaces to dissolve dissociative barriers, address relational ruptures, and cross-translate across polarizing tensions of difference. Enlisting capacities for collaborative meaning-making and interpersonal recognition, and drawing on empathy, imagination, and emotional expansion, the authors demonstrate how psychoanalytic practice can foster healing in communities navigating complex social and political challenges.

Essential reading for psychoanalysts, psychotherapists, and mental health professionals, this volume also guides students and scholars in applying psychoanalytic presence to urgent contemporary challenges, including social fragmentation, political polarization, and ecological crisis.

Johanna Dobrich, LCSW, is a New York City-based psychoanalyst, teacher, supervisor, and clinician specializing in the treatment of complex trauma and dissociative disorders. She teaches and consults widely, exploring relational dynamics, dissociation, and attachment. Johanna is the author of *Working with Survivor Siblings in Psychoanalysis* (2021) and recipient of the 2023 ISSTD Sandor Ferenczi Award.

PSYCHOANALYSIS IN A NEW KEY BOOK SERIES
DONNEL STERN
Series Editor

When music is played in a new key, the melody does not change, but the notes that make up the composition do: change in the context of continuity, continuity that perseveres through change. Psychoanalysis in a New Key publishes books that share the aims psychoanalysts have always had, but that approach them differently. The books in the series are not expected to advance any particular theoretical agenda, although to this date most have been written by analysts from the Interpersonal and Relational orientations.

The most important contribution of a psychoanalytic book is the communication of something that nudges the reader's grasp of clinical theory and practice in an unexpected direction. Psychoanalysis in a New Key creates a deliberate focus on innovative and unsettling clinical thinking. Because that kind of thinking is encouraged by exploration of the sometimes surprising contributions to psychoanalysis of ideas and findings from other fields, Psychoanalysis in a New Key particularly encourages interdisciplinary studies. Books in the series have married psychoanalysis with dissociation, trauma theory, sociology, and criminology. The series is open to the consideration of studies examining the relationship between psychoanalysis and any other field—for instance, biology, literary and art criticism, philosophy, systems theory, anthropology, and political theory.

But innovation also takes place within the boundaries of psychoanalysis, and Psychoanalysis in a New Key therefore also presents work that reformulates thought and practice without leaving the precincts of the field. Books in the series focus, for example, on the significance of personal values in psychoanalytic practice, on the complex interrelationship between the analyst's clinical work and personal life, on the consequences for the clinical situation when patient and analyst are from different cultures, and on the need for psychoanalysts to accept the degree to which they knowingly satisfy their own wishes during treatment hours, often to the patient's detriment.

A full list of all titles in this series is available at:
https://www.routledge.com/Psychoanalysis-in-a-New-Key-Book-Series/book-series/LEAPNKBS

Moving from Grievance to Hope in Psychoanalysis

Applied Case Studies

Edited by Johanna Dobrich

Routledge
Taylor & Francis Group
LONDON AND NEW YORK

Designed cover image: © Johanna Dobrich

First published 2027
by Routledge
4 Park Square, Milton Park, Abingdon, Oxon OX14 4RN

and by Routledge
605 Third Avenue, New York, NY 10158

Routledge is an imprint of the Taylor & Francis Group, an informa business

British Library Cataloguing-in-Publication Data
A catalogue record for this book is available from the British Library

ISBN: 978-1-041-11123-8 (hbk)
ISBN: 978-1-041-11040-8 (pbk)
ISBN: 978-1-003-65838-2 (ebk)

DOI: 10.4324/9781003658382

Typeset in Times New Roman
by SPi Technologies India Pvt Ltd (Straive)

For Lilah, whose spirit brings light to the night.
For Fegia Bine, whose loving and leading reach across time and space.
For my family, who share me with my writing, again and again.

Contents

Introduction

From Extremism to Intersubjectivity: Applied Psychoanalysis in Social Contexts

Johanna Dobrich

Developmental Psychoanalysis

Contemporary psychoanalysis is not just a modality of treatment but also a developmental perspective that accounts for the complexities inherent in humans being human together. A developmental perspective emphasizes growth, change, and transformation over time, whether in individuals, relationships, systems, or societies. It considers how psychological, emotional, and relational capacities emerge, evolve, and are shaped by experience, in response to both internal and external conditions. Contemporary developmental psychoanalysis was first brought into focus in the two-person model that ultimately emerged out of the Middle School of Psychoanalysis[1] from the writings of Melanie Klein, W.R.B. Fairbairn, D. W. Winnicott, Wilfred Bion, and Heinz Kohut, which broadened our understanding of the unconscious to encompass the real relational inputs of the parent–baby dyad as the foundational template for subjectivity and intrapsychic life. Bowlby (1969), and later attachment-oriented psychoanalysis (Beebe & Lachmann, 2002; Fonagy et al., 2002), further refined our understanding of the relationship between early developmental experiences and our unique capacities for relatedness that emerge in later collective life, setting a foundation for what follows.

All psychoanalytic developmental approaches share a fundamental understanding: development is not an automatic linear progression, and symptoms are not simply problems to be eradicated. Rather, they serve as meaningful expressions and communications of disrupted growth, power imbalances, environmental violations, and unmet needs. A developmental lens recognizes and supports the potential for emotional development at any stage of life and notices what types of environments facilitate versus inhibit such growth. Psychoanalysis as a

DOI: 10.4324/9781003658382-1

method offers a specialized environment for getting development back on track through relational connection, enabling the emergence of new capacities for feeling, relating, symbolizing, and conveying both unconscious and conscious experience, within and between people. Sandler and Fonagy (2004) write, “The therapeutic action of psychoanalysis involves not only uncovering unconscious material but also facilitating developmental changes in the patient’s capacity to mentalize and regulate affect within the therapeutic relationship” (p. 5), and I would add, beyond. Thus, developmental psychoanalysis illuminates how unmet developmental needs extend beyond the individual, shaping and reflecting collective and societal dynamics that demand therapeutic attention.

Psychoanalysis has long served as a powerful framework to uphold the ideals of dignity and self-sovereignty, particularly within discussions of social justice and identity. Psychoanalysis is a devoted practice dedicated to the emancipation of subjectivity. In recent times, across a broad spectrum of theoretical writings, psychoanalytic concepts have been invoked to articulate the psychological underpinnings of interdependent autonomy, human agency, and human worth.[2] These works underscore the importance of recognizing the intrapsychic and interpersonal impact of oppression, trauma, and resistance on a subject. However, despite this rich theoretical engagement, there remains a notable gap in the literature when it comes to the translation of these ideas into communal-based interventions.[3] Few scholars have undertaken the challenge of demonstrating just how psychoanalytic insights can be applied pragmatically to support developmental progression in real-world contexts, particularly those grappling with complex trauma and dissociation rooted in systemic relational violations.

This gap points to a pressing need for clinical scholarship that bridges theory and practice, offering tangible illustrations of how psychoanalytic principles can inform healing, resilience, and empowerment within diverse populations. Addressing this absence not only enriches psychoanalytic discourse but also advances its relevance and accessibility as a tool for meaningful social change. What is needed is a developmental lens that emphasizes transformation over time rather than static ideological formulations of causality and critique. This book seeks to address that imbalance by presenting a collection of case illustrations that demonstrate the expansive potential of applied psychoanalysis in contexts where grievance, struggle, and collective harm are pervasive.

Applied Psychoanalysis

Applied contemporary psychoanalysis provides a framework for understanding social and cultural phenomena that extends beyond individual treatment. This work entails the deployment of psychoanalytic concepts and methods to engage with and illuminate fields beyond the clinical setting, such as anthropology, religion, history, medicine, social justice, the arts, education, and public policy (Akhtar & Twemlow, 2020). The perspective offered here is that the mind is fundamentally relational and shaped by the dynamic interplay between individuals and their environments. A contemporary psychoanalytic view reveals that when ideology replaces relationality, a society's intrapsychic, interpersonal, and collective struggles become entrenched and inhibited. Ideology functions to maintain and justify power structures, social relations, and cultural norms, whereas relationality engages the dynamic, reciprocal nature of human interactions, and challenges the notion of the isolated, autonomous individual by foregrounding subjectivity as co-created through sustained engagement.[4] We are never outside ideology, yet placing our ideological commitments in a living dialectic with relationality provides a corrective to the excesses of any extreme (Guralnik & Simeon, 2010). When relationality is overemphasized, we may struggle to hold a position of our own. Whereas when ideology is overemphasized, we risk losing contact with the other's humanity, objectifying them in service of our ideological stance.

Relationality too, can be seen as a continuum that begins with affective permeability, where the self, molded by nonverbal exchanges and the subtle emotional currents of the caregiving environment, first comes into relation. At one end lies nonreflective relationally driven behavior, signaling a lack of relational sophistication, at the other the potential for intersubjectivity, where the self and other may be held in mutual recognition despite difference and tension (Mitchell, 2000). It is through these I–Thou moments that subjectivity is formed dialogically rather than independently (Stern, 2017). Intersubjectivity describes conditions in which mutual recognition and a capacity for shared meaning-making are possible within, between, and across subjects (Benjamin, 2004; Mitchell, 2000). It is a relational achievement, not a given. Since relationality exists on a continuum, it is subject to regressive and progressive variations within individuals and throughout time. The collision of various political contexts with the social collective may enhance or diminish the accessibility of intersubjective relating to groups and individuals, profoundly altering what is within reach. In other words, the developmental environment is not always conducive to the emergence of intersubjective relating, and some individuals, communities, or contexts may never have supported such relational capacities absent targeted intervention. This developmental scaffolding and skill building occurs within a medium psychoanalysts refer to as "the field." I argue that social psychoanalysis has a role to play in moving what is nonreflective[5] and automatic within individuals/groups back into a universe of possible shared meaning-making and mutual witnessing. Formulating and symbolizing affects such as rage, shame, paranoia, sadism, grief, and masochism is the work of the psychoanalysis. This is developmental work at a group level.

In recent years, the cultural milieu has undergone a discernible shift, diminishing our capacity to meet subjective complexity with curiosity and an openness to contradiction. Instead, social discourse has increasingly mirrored a kind of complementary warfare centering cause over relational engagement, in which dominant narratives vie for hegemonic authority through strategies of shame and moral absolutism, leaving little room for nuance, ambivalence, or dialogic growth (Benjamin, 2004). This shift within the environment has reduced the focus on relationality, favoring reactive stances that prioritize immediate response over reflective engagement and potential connection. Seeking relief from real moral injury through the objectification of others results in a corrosive feedback loop, where shame is amplified, forestalling the advancement of developmental progression that might otherwise lead to relational connection. The silencing of some subjective realties and the ossification of subjects into objects results in a proliferation of sadomasochistic struggles. This environmental slide into extreme polarization is pervasive and felt everywhere, even within our own discipline, where we are tasked with remaining reflective, active witnesses to multiplicity and their collisions.[6] Extremist ideology of *any* orientation or persuasion is not intersubjective in that it has already limited the scope of the problem to the "other," collapsing a space in which intersubjective awareness may be accessed. Extremism is defined as "the belief that an in-group's success or survival can never be separated from the need for hostile action against an out-group" (Berger, 2018, p. 155). Applied psychoanalysis offers a valuable lens through which to assess the emotional and relational dynamics within the field itself, enabling targeted interventions that address extremist influences, reduce polarization, and promote the emergence of a field capable of offering meaningful engagement across subjects.

The impetus for this book transpired from a conference I hosted at the Institute for Contemporary Psychotherapy in February 2025. In my opening remarks at the event, I offered three related ideas to support this initiative:

1 **Psychoanalysis as a field of study has increasingly become integrated with other disciplines such as social theory, neuroscience, and cultural studies**. This cross fertilization has led to new understandings of how unconscious processes shape not only individual but collective behavior and societal structures. It follows that contemporary psychoanalysis has something important to contribute in cultivating and supporting psychosocial development in flexible and adaptive directions.
2 **The social crises we face today challenge us to develop healing modalities that extend beyond the therapeutic dyad**. In the face of today's complex social and political climate, many clinicians feel a growing urgency to extend therapeutic insights beyond the consulting room and into the broader social world. Psychoanalysis has begun to take on a more activist role by modifying the analyst's identity and shifting the analytic frame to engage more flexibly with social and communal contexts (Echegoyen, 2022). The shift reflects both ethical responsibility and the understanding that individual psychic health is inseparable from social and relational contexts. Twemlow (2013) persuasively argues psychoanalysis has a central role to play in helping communities reorganize themselves psychologically and socially, by engaging psychoanalytic thinking in schools, homeless shelters, clinics, social service institutions, and more. Herman's (2023) recent work underscores that healing trauma extends beyond individual therapy, requiring transformation at the community, institutional, and societal levels.

3 **Narrativizing the effects of psychoanalytic interventions in restoring communal connection offers profound emotional value, helping us process despair, confusion, helplessness, anger, and pain, emotions central to modern life**. Storytelling becomes both a therapeutic practice and a meaningful end in itself, guiding individuals and communities from vicarious traumatization toward post-traumatic growth. In climates of widespread distress, uncertainty, and rapidly shifting political and social norms, the ability to manage our shared vulnerability well as clinicians is crucial. When societies are given the tools to articulate experiences of rupture through testimony, storytelling, and cultural expression, they engage in a form of collective psychic containment. These narratives act as vital psychic medicine, interrupting the hardening of defenses and the constriction that trauma produces. By making painful and dislocating experiences thinkable and shared, storytelling prevents emotional rigidity and invites compassion, reflection, and collective learning. This process nurtures the capacity to bear suffering with openness, enabling communities and us as clinicians, to transform trauma and adversity into resilience, insight, and meaningful growth.

The Unit of Analysis

The locus of analysis for applied psychoanalysis is very often the same place in which the work transpires—the field itself. Understanding the field as a complex system draws attention to the interplay between our inner psychic life and the social world, enriching both clinical work and social engagement. The concept of the field in psychoanalysis has evolved significantly over the past century, transforming in tandem with the shift from a one-person model to a contemporary, relational, systemic, and contextual understanding of psychic life. Bion (1962) articulated a vision of the analytic "field" as a theoretical construct referring to the total psychological-emotional environment of the analytic encounter. This "field" shapes and is shaped by the experiences of both analyst and patient, making the therapeutic setting a living system that influences the unfolding of the analytic process. Ogden (1986, 1994), Harris (1997), Baranger and Baranger (2008), Bollas (1987), and Stolorow and Atwood (1992) each elaborated on a feature of the analytic field—the third space it generates—between patient and analyst as a dynamic, co-created relational environment in which meaning, emotion, and transformation emerge collaboratively. But this view of the field extends far beyond the immediate therapeutic relationship, encompassing a complex, dynamic system that integrates sociocultural, historical, and environmental factors, underscoring how these broader social realities both influence and are influenced by the psychoanalytic process.

The "field" is now seen not only as a metaphor but also as a clinical reality: a dynamic, co-created relational space that holds unspoken truths, collective memory, and emotional resonance. Therapists regularly intervene at the level of individual insight, as well as at the level of the field, attuning to and shifting it through presence, relational stance, and contextual awareness. Stern (2017) writes, "The analytic field is a co-constructed, intersubjective matrix in which analyst and patient are enmeshed. It is a dynamic and fluid space where unconscious communications, enactments, and emotional truths emerge and are experienced jointly, transcending a simple two-person or one-person psychology" (p. 3). While the field is primarily the shared psychological space within therapy, Stern acknowledges its permeability to, and formation by, external social and cultural influences. This intersubjective perspective implies that efforts to address social problems without attending to the relational and contextual field in which they arise risk becoming mechanistic and formulaic rather than engaging with the creative, dynamic process necessary for meaningful transformation. Psychoanalysts are trained to attune to environments as much as they are to individual psyches. Arguably, social psychoanalysis treats the field itself as the patient, working to reveal its subjective experience and to foster cohesion and development.

This book represents a sample of educator-clinicians who navigate the balance between individual practice and collective engagement across a wide array of social issues. Each in their own way is listening and working with the field in their interventions. Importantly, each contributor moves beyond using psychoanalytic theory simply to interpret and describe social crises. They also illustrate, through real-world examples, how they shifted the focus toward reestablishing intersubjectivity and pluralism, which are hallmarks of a healthy collective endeavor. Pluralism relies on valuing differentiated subjectivities, relational negotiation, while preserving the autonomy of distinct perspectives to a degree. It does not require consensus or uniformity, even though not all positions may be equally sophisticated or emancipatory, distinguishing it from models that aim to suppress difference or enforce hegemonic conformity. In pluralism, engaging with difference and negotiating consensus are ongoing relational processes that preserve the integrity of each subjectivity while fostering cooperation across distinctions (Slavin & Kriegman, 1998). One cannot reduce an "opponent" to an Other if their engagement or participation is necessary to build coalitions and effect meaningful change. These educator-clinicians offer inspiring examples of how they have integrated psychoanalytic interventions in social spaces.

One of the greatest challenges we face in present day collective life is breaking out of a paranoid-schizoid mode of relatedness, which encourages a zero-sum view of the world, rigid defenses, and extremist solutions (Ogden, 1986). This perspective reinforces binary thinking, making it seem like supporting one cause requires opposing another, and this polarized stance moves through groups like contagion. Benjamin (2004) refers to this as a climate of complementarity, a structural relation where one party can only view the other/s in objectifying terms. Developmental psychoanalysis teaches us that extreme polarization signals a disruption in healthy social development and a failure to mentalize the totality of the field. Such polarization collapses imaginative space and exposes an obedience to the limiting belief that needed internal objects demand only our submission rather than our full engagement.

In community settings, complementarity is not something we diagnose from a distance but something we inevitably find ourselves inside of. Power asymmetries whether they be professional, institutional, racial, economic, or otherwise, shape the relational field, and naming them explicitly becomes the first gesture toward loosening the doer/done-to dynamic (Benjamin, 2004). Rather than relying on the safety of the expert stance, community psychoanalysts turn toward lateral models of shared knowing, recognizing that communities hold their own forms of wisdom and survival knowledge (Dobrich & Saidipour, in press). Community psychoanalysts act as facilitators and translators. Enactments become understood not as missteps but as meaningful communications: repetitions of injuries asking to be acknowledged in a communal space. Psychoanalysts can help communities resist collapsing into simple binaries of victim and aggressor, or helper and helped, and instead make space for the complexity, variety and ambivalence that characterize all human encounters. Out of this mutual risking emerges the possibility of thirdness, a jointly created relational space in which multiple parties can recognize one another as subjects (Benjamin, 2004). Applied psychoanalysis engages environments marked by complementarity, opening developmental pathways to deeper connection and shared understanding.

Framework for Engagement

This book unfolds across nine chapters, each engaging with different applications of contemporary psychoanalysis in relation to sociopolitical life and emotional development. Drawing on clinical material, theoretical perspectives, and cultural analysis, the chapters explore how psychoanalytic thinking and practice can respond to, and shape, collective experience, tilting it on a developmental trajectory toward growth. With this in mind, I invite you to engage with each chapter while holding the specifics lightly. Listen beneath the particular examples to sense what recurs across cases. Depth emerges when we attend to process rather than content, revealing the structure of subjectivity and intersubjectivity, or its absence.

Grievance is best understood as a developmental trauma response to one's subjective experience being annihilated or under threat over long periods of time by a perceived uncaring other(s) or culture. When people feel that their experience is not held, the reptilian brain takes over to manage this threat of psychological and/or physical erasure or domination. The reptilian responses are not consciously chosen and include fight, flight, freeze, fawn, and collapse. However, none of these states of being can manage complexity, as they are only meant to help an organism sustain life in the face of threat. If a person, group, or culture is locked into a state of perpetual grievance, then the hope of intersubjective recognition and healthy attachments to others remains out of reach, not only because of the host culture's limitations but also because the internal structure of the aggrieved is developmentally stuck.

Consider these questions:

- How do psychoanalysts use their listening stance and participation to impact the field and create environmental conditions that allow for possibilities to emerge among cohorts?
- How does the function of holding at the social level impact the psychic experience within collective functioning?
- How do we conceptualize moving groups from a paranoid-schizoid position of scarcity, binary thinking, and extremism—common emotional responses to social trauma—into a depressive position that allows for movement, imagination, expansion, and new coalitions of meaning-making to emerge?
- What do each of these cases have in common?
- What do these cases illuminate about the process of moving from grievance to hope, while still preserving the psychological and symbolic utility of socially identifications?

Extremism and the Echoes of Injury

Extremism defines culpability rather than discovering it and reflects an early mode of relationality. In contrast, intersubjective relating requires a tolerance for uncertainty—a dropping of ego-driven, self-protective behavior—and looks to both deficits and potentialities across subjects. If intersubjective relating requires a continual reckoning of self with the Other, grievance assumes one already knows oneself and the offender in a fixed way. Berger (2018) defines grievance as

> more than a momentary feeling of discontent or a short-lived, even explosive expression of anger or frustration; rather it is a conclusion reached about the reason for the offender's suffering (or the suffering of others about whom the offender cares): it is a function of concreteness- a tangible, identifiable object to which causation of suffering can be ascribed.
>
> (p. 130)

The capacity to listen and to be moved or transformed through relational engagement requires a field that is open to inquiry and supported by developmental scaffolding. It is much harder than staking a position and determining a priori what things mean and requires the evolution of maturational experience. The paranoid-schizoid notion of alleviating grievance relies on power reversals as the solution to injuries rooted in powerlessness or hopelessness, but this undeveloped and incomplete perspective cannot respond to the complexity of our modern problems. Many today carry multiple identifications—as both marginalized and marginalizers, and privileged and socially disadvantaged—in different proportions that vary by context. To promote psychological healing for the collective, you need to know how to transmute shame, petrification, anger, and loss in individuals. Additionally, you need to facilitate the foreclosed mourning held by those who are stuck in aggrievement (Ogden, 1986). Relocating shame from one group to another is not effective. Grievance limits "capacities to see the world and other people more fully or to see many different parts of oneselves as fully as possible" (Greene & Brodbar, 2010, p. 316).

A redistribution of resources—be they economic, political, social, or emotional—on its own would not suffice to alter the trajectory of persecutory experience. The medium in which experience is generated must be changed too. Justice, defined here as equitable access to resources, cannot be predetermined, predefined, and actualized for some at the expense of the other, whoever that other happens to be, or it fails to promote intersubjective relationality. In this framework, justice is conceived as a process of social repair that unfolds within the relational field of community response and recognition, not through punitive interventions (Herman, 2023). Ideologies of grievance can either clash and come to heads for the moral majority in extremist battles, or they can be revealed as incomplete stories we tell ourselves as we swim into the unchartered developmental waters of a truly intersubjective exchange that promises to mature and ripen us even as it changes us along the way.

It is a particular skill of dissociation-informed psychoanalysts to move a patient from a state of chronic disempowerment and grievance into security, connection, and a capacity, in Ogden's terms, for depressive positionality and relationality, where integration, ambivalence, conflict, and contradiction become tolerable (Benjamin, 2004; Ogden, 1986). These are precursors to intersubjective relating in which a present subject becomes embodied to hold and process unexperienced experience, allowing for genuine presence rather than reactive responses to life (Dobrich, 2021). We need models of identity and collectivity that embrace complexity, not models that locate the problem entirely outside the self/group thereby perpetuating conditions of disempowerment and zero-sum thinking that prevent the emergence out of despair in the future.

Drawing on Layton (2007), we can see that while social norms limit the psychic positions we can occupy, identity formation is fundamentally ambivalent: it can be a source of trauma, yet it also holds the potential to generate transformative and emancipatory forms of subjectivity. The case studies illuminated in this volume demonstrate how psychoanalysts embrace complexity and guide communities in tolerating a full range of affect. They offer alternatives to frameworks that externalize problems and perpetuate disempowerment and mutually exclusive thinking. In doing so, these narratives foster pathways out of despair, toward resilience, reflection, and post-traumatic growth.

Making Meaning with Applied Psychoanalysis: A Map of What Follows

Psychoanalysis teaches us that truth is neither wholly objective nor predetermined; rather, it is always in the process of becoming epistemologically grasped, shaped profoundly by the intersection of subjectivities. Hart writes (2021/2022), "Radical openness involves a disciplined psychoanalytic stance of attempting to notice, question, and relinquish presumptions about oneself and the other." It follows that environments that promote a greater tendency toward reflection over reaction are qualitatively necessary for psychological growth. This book draws on psychoanalytic theory not merely as a lens to illuminate the unconscious and emotional undercurrents shaping our contemporary socio-political landscape—including the healing of refugees (Chapter 1), the plight of war-torn and traumatized children (Chapter 2), the reckoning with legacies of racism and erasure (Chapter 3), the navigation of inter-ethnic conflict (Chapter 4), the articulation of maternal identity and embodiment (Chapter 5), the challenge of American gun violence (Chapter 6), the educational needs of asylum-seeking and disabled children (Chapter 7), the shadows of ethnocultural internalized self-hatred and self-erasure (Chapter 8), and the witness of environmental degradation (Chapter 9)—but also as a vital mode of intervention.

By shifting the locus of intervention from the individual to the surrounding relational and environmental field, and by working to alter the very medium in which psychic life unfolds, this approach advances a model of clinical praxis oriented toward relational repair. In doing so, it articulates an ethic of care that extends beyond the confines of the consulting room and engages the sociopolitical world as a necessary site of psychoanalytic attention (Echegoyen, 2022).

Notes

1 The "middle school" refers to a transitional period in psychoanalytic history, roughly from the 1930s to the 1960s, during which theorists expanded the field beyond Freud's biologically driven instinct model to include a greater emphasis on real relationships, the self, and developmental processes (Mitchell & Aron, 1999).

2 For example, Ahmed (2000), Benjamin (1988), Butler (1990), Drescher (1998), Eng and Han (2003), Fanon (1952), Frosh (2002), Sedgwick (1990), Sue (2010), and Echegoyen (2022) offer incisive cultural critiques that interrogate foundational assumptions of psychoanalytic thought in order to illuminate its limitations in meeting social problems/specific communities. However, their efforts have emphasized theoretical frameworks, with community-based applications still emerging.

3 An important notable example of linking psychoanalytic ideas with direct social intervention in a group context is the recent Holmes Commission on Racial Equality in American Psychoanalysis *Final Report*, published by the American Psychoanalytic Association in 2023, which offers institutional corrective measures to address racial injury going beyond theory into policy actions.

4 Althusser (1971) argues that ideology produces subjects through the mechanism of *interpellation*, in which individuals are "hailed" into social positions (pp. 170–177).

5 From a contemporary relational perspective, nonreflective actions are not viewed as instinct driven but instead as shaped by the ongoing interplay between subjectivity and real relational experiences. These actions are unreflective not because they are primitive but because they have not yet been brought into awareness.

6 For example, on May 25, 2025, President Stephen Soldz of Division 39 of the APA resigned suddenly, stating in a personal communication:

> I had hoped to facilitate a division open to new sociopolitical perspectives on the intrapsychic while building upon more traditional psychoanalytic work of theory and technique {but} there are deep schisms on the board about what that direction ought to be, and I have not been able to bridge them.

References

Ahmed, S. (2000). *Strange encounters: Embodied others in post-coloniality*. Routledge.

Akhtar, S., & Twemlow, S. W. (Eds.). (2020). *Textbook of applied psychoanalysis*. Routledge. https://doi.org/10.4324/9781003076223

Althusser, L. (1971). Ideology and ideological state apparatuses (notes towards an investigation). In *Lenin and philosophy and other essays* (B. Brewster, Trans., pp. 127–186). Monthly Review Press.

Baranger, M., & Baranger, W. (2008). The analytic situation as a dynamic field. *The International Journal of Psychoanalysis*, *89*(4), 795–826. https://doi.org/10.1111/j.1745-8315.2008.00074.x

Beebe, B., & Lachmann, F. (2002). Infant research and adult treatment: Co-constructing interactions. *Psychoanalytic Dialogues*, *12*(5), 629–654. https://doi.org/10.4324/9780203767498

Benjamin, J. (1988). *The bonds of love: Psychoanalysis, feminism, and the problem of domination*. Pantheon Books.

Benjamin, J. (2004). Beyond doer and done to: An intersubjective view of thirdness. *The Psychoanalytic Quarterly*, *73*(1), 5–46.

Berger, J. M. (2018). *Extremism*. The MIT Press.

Bion, W. R. (1962). *Learning from experience*. Heinemann.

Bollas, C. (1987). *The shadow of the object: Psychoanalysis of the unthought known*. Free Association Books.

Bowlby, J. (1969). *Attachment and loss: Vol. 1. Attachment*. Basic Books.

Butler, J. (1990). *Gender trouble: Feminism and the subversion of identity*. Routledge.

Dobrich, J. (2021). *Working with survivor siblings in psychoanalysis: Ability and disability in clinical process*. Routledge.

Dobrich, J., & Saidipour, P. (in press). Got milk?: A lateral tale of formulating our socio-cultural identities in psychoanalytic supervision. *Contemporary Psychoanalysis*.

Drescher, J. (Ed.). (1998). *Psychoanalytic therapy and the gay man*. Routledge.

Echegoyen, R. (2022). Abandoning the analytic frame. *Division Review*, *28* (Winter 2022), 28–30.

Eng, D. L., & Han, S. (2003). Racial melancholia, racial dissociation: On the social and psychic lives of Asian Americans. *Psychoanalytic Dialogues*, *13*(1), 1–27.

Fanon, F. (1952). *Black skin, white masks* (C. L. Markmann, Trans.). Grove Press. (Original work published 1952).

Fonagy, P., Gergely, G., Jurist, E. L., & Target, M. (2002). *Affect regulation, mentalization, and the development of the self*. Other Press.

Frosh, S. (2002). *Psychoanalysis and social justice: Perspectives on the study of subjectivity*. Palgrave Macmillan.

Greene, B., & Brodbar, D. (2010). A minyan of women: Family dynamics, Jewish identity and psychotherapy practice. *Women & Therapy*, *33*(3–4), 155–157. https://doi.org/10.1080/02703141003766282

Guralnik, O., & Simeon, D. (2010). Depersonalization: Standing in the spaces between recognition and interpellation. *Psychoanalytic Dialogues*, *20*(4), 400–416. https://doi.org/10.1080/10481885.2010.502501

Harris, A. (1997). *The analytic field*. Routledge.

Hart, A. H. (2021/2022). *From multicultural competence to radical openness: A psychoanalytic engagement of otherness*. https://apsa.org/wp-content/uploads/apsaa-publications/vol51no1-TOC/html/vol51no1_09.xhtml

Herman, J. L. (2023). *Truth and repair: How trauma survivors envision justice*. Basic Books.

Layton, L. (2007). What psychoanalysis, culture and society mean to me. *Mens Sana Monographs*, *5*(1), 146–157.

Mitchell, S. A. (2000). *Relationality: From attachment to intersubjectivity*. Routledge.

Mitchell, S. A., & Aron, L. (1999). *Relational psychoanalysis: The emergence of a tradition*. Analytic Press.

Ogden, T. H. (1986). *The matrix of the mind: Object relations and the psychoanalytic dialogue*. Jason Aronson.

Ogden, T. H. (1994). The analytic third: Working with intersubjective clinical facts. *The International Journal of Psycho-Analysis*, *75*, 3–19.

Sandler, J., & Fonagy, P. (2004). Developmental perspectives on the therapeutic action of psychoanalysis. *International Journal of Psychoanalysis*, *85*(1), 1–14.

Sedgwick, E. K. (1990). *Epistemology of the closet*. University of California Press.

Slavin, M. O., & Kriegman, D. (1998). Why the analyst needs to change: Toward a theory of conflict, negotiation, and mutual influence in the therapeutic process. *Psychoanalytic Dialogues*, *8*(2), 247–284. https://doi.org/10.1080/10481889809539246

Stern, D. B. (2017). *On the analytic field*. Routledge.

Stolorow, R. D., & Atwood, G. E. (1992). *Contexts of being: The intersubjective foundations of psychological life*. Analytic Press.

Sue, D. W. (2010). *Microaggressions in everyday life: Race, gender, and sexual orientation*. Wiley.

Twemlow, S. W. (2013). Broadening the vision: A case for community-based psychoanalysis in the context of usual practice. *Journal of the American Psychoanalytic Association*, *61*(4), 663–690.

Chapter 1

Beyond Borders

Psychoanalytic Perspectives on Refugee Healing

Ruth Wyatt and Alexander Beznes

Introduction: A Call to Action

Historically, psychoanalysis has been rooted in the one-on-one encounter between analyst and patient within the confines of the treatment room, emphasizing the internal world of the individual. This model was long considered foundational to psychoanalytic practice. Although there were some early efforts to broaden its reach through community-based clinics, politically engaged projects, and a philosophy of science exploring unconscious experience and human motivation, these initiatives remained exceptions rather than the norm and were marginalized. Freud's own stance reflects this tension. While he defended the legitimacy of lay analysis and expressed hope that psychoanalysis might become more widely accessible, the early movement remained largely restrictive in both theory and practice. In *The Question of Lay Analysis* (Freud, 1926/1990), he argued that psychoanalysis should not be limited to medical doctors, emphasizing its concern with psychic life rather than somatic disease. He also supported free clinics such as the Vienna Ambulatorium, which aimed to bring treatment to the working class. Yet Freud remained cautious about broad democratization, fearing that poorly trained practitioners might dilute the discipline. As Jacoby (1983) and Kirsner (2000) have shown, he distanced himself from followers like Wilhelm Reich and Otto Fenichel, who sought to align psychoanalysis with socialist and community-based movements. Thus, Freud's position was marked by contradiction: he articulated a vision of psychoanalysis as universally applicable yet participated in and reinforced structures that kept it largely within bourgeois, professional, and Eurocentric circles.

DOI: 10.4324/9781003658382-2

By the mid-20th century, politically engaged psychoanalysts were further pushed to the margins. As Layton (2006) and Jacoby (1983) argue, psychoanalysis gradually turned inward, focusing closely on the clinical frame, which inadvertently excluded large segments of the population. Working with displaced individuals, the poor, and people of color was viewed as compromising conditions necessary for analytic rigor. However, over time, the impact of this limited focus on the frame and analytic rigor has become readily evident, particularly in relation to collective trauma and structural inequalities.

In recent decades, the field has begun to shift. Developments in trauma theory, intersubjectivity, and cultural studies have reoriented psychoanalysis toward an appreciation of the social context. The analytic third is increasingly seen not only as a shared psychic space but also as one shaped by history, embodiment, and asymmetries of power (Altman, 1993; Orange, 2016). Global crises such as mass displacement, racial injustice, and the COVID-19 pandemic have only deepened this turn toward the sociopolitical (Boulanger & Rosenberg, 2023; Hollander, 2010; Margherita & Tessitore, 2023).

This shift is evident in initiatives like the Holmes Commission on Racial Equality in American Psychoanalysis (Holmes et al., 2024), the film *Black Psychoanalysts Speak* (Winograd, 2014), and Neil Altman's long-standing work on poverty and access to care (Altman, 1993). It is also reflected globally in programs such as Brazil's public mental health clinics (Minozzo & Soreanu, 2024), France's La Borde clinic (Oury, 2024), and Argentinian community psychoanalysis (Onofrio & Kitroser, 2021). These efforts reimagine psychoanalysis as a tool for both individual healing and social repair.

Within this broader reorientation, psychoanalysis is beginning to reclaim its early capacity to link individual experience with collective rupture. Programs like the Refugee Support Program (RSP) do not simply apply analytic concepts to new populations; they challenge us to rethink what constitutes analytic work in the first place. They invite us to understand communities as psychic entities (Ainslie, 2017), trauma as both intrapsychic and geopolitical, and healing as a relational and ethical act that occurs not only between two people in a room but also across networks of care, solidarity, and social repair.

This chapter explores the psychoanalytic dimensions of refugee trauma and clinical and collective response through three interwoven threads: (1) trauma theory, as described earlier; (2) the applied psychoanalytic framework of the RSP; and (3) the clinical case of Macey, a Ukrainian refugee whose journey brings these dynamics to life. Together, these threads demonstrate how psychoanalysis—when expanded beyond the consulting room—can speak to the psychic, cultural, and political fractures of our time.

Applied Psychoanalysis: The Refugee Support Program

The RSP, housed within the Psychoanalytic Psychotherapy Study Center (PPSC), a New York City–based psychoanalytic training institute, stands among the contemporary efforts to bring psychoanalysis into active engagement with healing individual and collective trauma. Initiated in response to the mental health crisis following the war in Ukraine in February 2022 by Board Member Viktor Diugunovych and Founding Director Judy Levitz, RSP was launched to meet a direct social need from *within* a psychoanalytic training program. The program began by mobilizing licensed clinicians to offer one to five Zoom sessions as volunteer trauma counselors, with the option to refer clients for longer-term care. But the needs quickly outpaced this original scope. Drawing lessons from earlier crises like 9/11 and Hurricane Sandy, RSP expanded its model to include five core areas: clinical care, asylum advocacy, translation and care coordination, resettlement support, and clinician training.

Since its founding, RSP has provided services to more than 1,000 individuals and currently provides help to 180 Ukrainians in the United States and in Ukraine. Its infrastructure depends on more than 80 volunteers, including clinicians, translators, asylum advocates, care coordinators, research liaisons, and administrative staff—who together sustain a dynamic, multi-layered system of care. All clinicians are vetted and supported by trauma-informed workshops and supervision groups hosted by PPSC. As such, RSP offers a model for extending psychoanalytic thinking into the larger world, bridging therapeutic practice with community-based response. It brings analytic thought to bear not only on psychic suffering but also on the systemic conditions, legal precarity, cultural dislocation, and communal rupture that shape and sustain trauma. Through its integration of clinical services, clinician training, community partnerships, and legal advocacy, RSP operationalizes a form of psychoanalysis that is both relational and reparative, rooted in healing and solidarity.

Refugee Trauma as Psychosocial Crisis

Since the war in Ukraine began in February 2022, more than 7 million people have fled the country, with an additional 3.7 million internally displaced. Approximately 240,000 Ukrainians have resettled in the United States (Statista, 2025). These numbers reflect not only a humanitarian emergency but also a psychological rupture that spans both individual and collective dimensions.

The trauma of forced displacement is never purely individual. While it registers deeply in the psychic life of the refugee, its origins are political, systemic, and collective. This section explores how such trauma takes shape both within the individual and across communities and how psychoanalysis, while historically focused on the inner world, is increasingly called to respond to these wider ruptures.

The trauma experienced by refugees is profound and complex. It often begins with the violent uprooting from home and country, an experience rooted not only in personal loss but also in geopolitical conflict and the breakdown of collective structures. Displacement and breakdown lead to disorientation and loss: unfamiliar environments, language barriers, and unemployment (Luci, 2020), and at times basic insecurity around food and shelter. Under such strain, refugees often live with persistent fear and looming uncertainty. In therapy with RSP clinicians, Ukrainian clients ask questions like: *Will I ever return home? Is my family safe? What is my future?* (A. Beznes, personal communication, April 10, 2025). These are not just logistical concerns; they are existential fractures.

Unprocessed trauma often manifests in states of dissociation, fear, and psychic rigidity. Melanie Klein's concept of the paranoid-schizoid position provides a useful lens here: when overwhelmed by anxiety, the ego splits experience into binaries—safe/dangerous, good/bad, us/them (Klein, 1946). In the wake of forced displacement, such early defenses can resurface, leading refugees to experience the external world as profoundly threatening and their inner world as fragmented (Akhtar, 1995). Symbolization and reflective capacity may be impaired, and affect remains unprocessed, expelled rather than metabolized (Alayarian, 2019).

This psychic splitting is not only an individual response but often mirrors the breakdown of collective structures that once held and contained meaning. When trauma cannot be contained and metabolized, it remains an unformulated experience (Bromberg, 1996; Stern, 1983) lodged in the psyche as fragmented memory and language. This disrupts the psychic function of reverie, which is the ability to reflect, imagine, and integrate experience, engendering continuity over time (Bryon, 2021). There is no past, present, or future when one is frozen in a state of trauma (Stern, 2017). The result is psychic fragmentation, a condition that afflicts both individuals and communities (Bryon, 2021).

Where verbal expression is not yet accessible, somatic symptoms often take its place. Additionally, trauma, at least initially, is often experienced as visual, olfactory, auditory, or kinesthetic sensations. The patient ultimately, with the clinician's help, must learn to tolerate and integrate these sensations so that they can put them into words that represent the narrative of *what happened* in order to be able to move forward (van der Kolk, 1994).

Refugee trauma reverberates through the communities in which displaced individuals reside—to the collective and social dimensions as well (Margherita & Tessitore, 2023). Communities function as "psychic entities" (Ainslie, 2017), offering essential psychological support by providing spaces in which members can feel held and sustained. When communities are lost or destroyed, the psychological impact on individuals can be profound. Thus, the reconstitution of community becomes a critical element in the healing process for those who have been displaced (Ainslie, 2017).

The Therapeutic Response: A Framework for Healing

If the refugee experience is characterized by isolation, voicelessness, and a paranoid-schizoid position, the therapeutic stance must address these specific wounds with intentional care and containment. The goal of therapy, then, is to create a reliable and containing environment that allows movement toward the *depressive position* where reverie and repair can take place. Here, the refugee begins to mourn what was lost, hold ambivalence, and tolerate the pain of mixed feelings, what Klein saw as essential to the capacity for integration (Klein, 1946). The depressive position, in turn, fosters a more cohesive sense of self and other, allowing the patient to reclaim a sense of continuity in the midst of rupture (Klein, 1946) and to participate in the creation or recreation of community. Healing, in this context, involves both psychological and communal repair, an aim that lies at the heart of RSP's mission. The program is not only structured to support individual transformation but also to rebuild fractured communal ties and facilitate participation in shared social life.

This type of healing requires attending to the following domains.

Restoring Voice and Narrative Continuity

One of the key tasks of therapy when working with refugees is to help organize traumatic experience into a coherent narrative, reconnecting past, present, and future. Part of this work is to help the refugee regain their voice to create space for speech where silence or fragmentation has reigned (Boulanger, 2008). In the presence of empathic attunement, the unspeakable becomes speakable, and the traumatic can be named and symbolized, and the patient can reclaim agency and identity (Bromberg, 1996; Stern, 1983). This act of voicing has implications well beyond the descriptive, eliciting transformations at both the individual and collective levels that create cohesiveness and deepened subjectivity within communal bonds (Stern, 1983). In RSP's model, restoring narrative coherence is not only a clinical task but also a socially reparative one, enabling the refugee to rejoin a community that recognizes their story, their loss, and their agency.

One of RSP's core aims is to create a "holding environment" where refugee clients can begin to process traumatic experiences within a safe, attuned therapeutic relationship (Alayarian, 2019). Clinicians are trained to tolerate intense affect, dissociation, and narrative incoherence, common features of trauma, while bearing witness to the client's psychic states. Central to this work is empathy, which, as Kohut emphasized, functions not only as a means of understanding but as a therapeutic action in its own right. He described empathy as "a therapeutic action in the broadest sense," highlighting its capacity to promote healing and restore self-cohesion (Kohut, 1981/2010, p. 554). To support this challenging work, RSP offers ongoing training to its clinicians in trauma theory, EMDR tapping, dialectical behavior therapy (DBT), cultural sensitivity, collective trauma, and embodied care. Specialized support is also extended to interpreters, who often navigate complex intersections of language, culture, and trauma.

Building an Intersubjective Relationship and Linking to Community

The mutuality born from the therapeutic relationship can foster the emergence of a collective identity, linking individual healing to broader communal restoration, re-embedding individuals into shared structures of meaning and support (Koh & Twemlow, 2018).

RSP's holistic model reflects this orientation, recognizing that rebuilding the external scaffolding of life such as housing, education, employment, and legal services can support the psychic processes of mourning and repair. Central to this mission are RSP's asylum advocates, who provide informed, compassionate support to their clients seeking asylum and navigating the legal system. These advocates have completed specialized training through the Weill Cornell Center for Human Rights and help guide clients through the complex asylum application process.

When refugees are connected to legal advocacy, social services, and community networks, the isolating effects of trauma and displacement begin to soften. In their place, a sense of solidarity emerges, one that unites both refugee and helper in a shared human experience. This collective dimension of healing validates suffering as a social and political condition rather than a private pathology (Kane, 2005). At RSP, practical and psychological needs are not treated as separate domains but as deeply interwoven expressions of survival, identity, and resilience.

Community-building efforts form a vital bridge between the individual treatment room and the wider collective. RSP fosters community among clients through a range of initiatives designed to promote connection, belonging, and shared experience. These include support groups and activity-based groups such as a film club for adults, as well as a children's music group and support group for children with physical and emotional disabilities (offered for clients in Ukraine). Community-building structures in New York include workshops, support groups, and communal events that emphasize mutual recognition and group cohesion.

One powerful example of RSP's community-based work is a pottery workshop and support group created by Alexander Beznes, a clinician and member of the RSP leadership team, specifically for refugees experiencing loneliness and identity loss following resettlement. The workshop, named Eyes Fear, Hands Do after a Slavic proverb, builds on a shared cultural foundation and channels the spirit of collective empowerment. Through the act of creation, participants connect with others who have faced similar ruptures, transforming solitude into solidarity. Artistic practice becomes a mode of psychic integration, what Rose (1990) describes as fostering "shifts in perspective" and restoring a "sense of wholeness."

Recognizing that therapeutic work with refugees often evokes profound emotional strain, RSP also attends to the needs of its clinicians. Vicarious trauma and compassion fatigue are common risks in crisis work (Saakvitne, 2002), and self-care is not viewed as ancillary but as essential. Ongoing supervision, training, and reflective practice are core components of RSP's model, offering clinicians spaces to process their experiences, metabolize emotional burdens, and sustain their capacity for empathic engagement. These spaces encourage therapists to engage with their own countertransference and cultural positioning. RSP's model of mutual attunement exemplifies this communal and relational space. In this way, the care RSP provides extends in all directions: from client to clinician, from individual to collective, from survival to restoration—and from psychic rupture to social repair.

Reclaiming Voice and Agency: Macey's Journey Toward Integration

This section is based on the work of Alexander Beznes, LCSW.

Macey sought psychological support in the fall of 2024 after enduring profound displacement in the aftermath of the full-scale invasion of Ukraine. When the war broke out, she was forced to take shelter in a basement with her husband and young daughter until it was safe to evacuate. Hearing explosions throughout the night left her feeling shaken and powerless, echoing the chaos of her parents arguing during her childhood. Fleeing her hometown and leaving the life she knew behind in Kharkiv—coupled with the uncertainty that she could ever return—upended her sense of stability and safety.

After a brief period of refuge in Eastern Europe, the family sought asylum in the United States to be closer to economic opportunities and eventually settled in a small northeastern town where her husband's cousin runs a business. Macey is faced with the daunting challenge of adjusting to life in a foreign land, learning a new language, and navigating a precarious immigration status. The escalating household tensions, collapsing boundaries, and deteriorating health of her family push her to the brink as she tries to hold onto a sense of hope amid a tenuous future.

Embodied Anxiety and a Fragmented Sense of Safety

When I began working with Macey, she was overwhelmed by debilitating anxiety after her mother-in-law's recent cancer diagnosis sent her family further into crisis. A local nonprofit had helped them get settled with their basic needs, such as healthcare benefits, when they first arrived, laying a stable foundation essential to trauma treatment (Zaleski et al., 2016). This latest setback threatened to disrupt the fragile sense of safety her family had only recently started to rebuild. It also resurfaced the trauma of a painful period when her husband had a serious health scare shortly after her father-in-law's death. Macey tearfully resonated with my interpretation that she had been carrying the emotional burden of her family's health issues, isolated in her pain as her husband grew emotionally absent due to his demanding job. She shared his observation that she does "everything for others and nothing for herself" as a way of regaining control amidst great uncertainty. The emotional toll of these traumatic events manifested as severe somatic distress such as acid reflux, tearfulness, and chronic tension that made her muscles feel like "stones." Macey reported feeling significantly "lighter" after finally giving voice to emotions long held in silence—the knot in her throat loosening and her breath expanding (Ogden et al., 2006).

Over the course of our work together, she would end particularly draining sessions saying that she felt like a "squeezed out lemon" or "rag," images that captured her exhaustion and relief. Bringing awareness to the tension held in her body, with the aim of developing mindfulness, was central to helping Macey reclaim a sense of agency and competence (van der Kolk, 2002). From this regulated state, she gradually found emotional release through somatic interventions that built interoceptive awareness (Fisher, 2015). However, it would be some time before Macey could let her guard down. She described feeling "fear in everything," paralyzed by the thought of "making a mistake." Since the onset of the war, Macey's life had been marked by hypervigilance and chronic worry, leading her to embody a paranoid-schizoid position in which the world felt "deeply threatening" (Alayarian, 2019).

Her fears were especially focused on her 7-year-old daughter, whose recurring illnesses and frequent school absences compounded her difficulties adjusting, making friends, and navigating a language barrier. Though time at home gave her more opportunities to connect and care for her, it also left her feeling trapped in her own anxious thoughts. Macey recognized that staying home deepened her depression by depriving her of the movement and stimulation she relied on to cope. Learning to shift out of this hypervigilant state toward rest and relaxation would prove to be one of the most enduring challenges in our work. Survivors of trauma often struggle to regulate their nervous systems, remaining caught in a persistent flight-or-fight response (van der Kolk, 2002).

Macey was becoming increasingly nervous ahead of her daughter's upcoming tonsil surgery. On a particularly restless night, she lay awake and monitored her daughter's congested breathing while she recovered from a cold. She described how the pauses in between her breaths felt intolerable to her, waking her up if she stopped breathing for too long. Macey was unraveling in response to all of the uncertainty in her life, becoming more hypervigilant and fearful. She recalled trying to journal about this experience, but seeing her thoughts on paper threatened to bring her worst fears to life. She ended up quickly crossing out her words, effectively nullifying their existence, unable to give voice to horrible imaginings.

Macey shared how she scrutinized the details of the appearance of her daughter's surgeon, trying to pick up on subtle cues in his appearance (e.g., fingernails, hair) to determine if he was trustworthy and competent. In retrospect, I felt fortunate that I had passed this level of scrutiny from her by being a calm and accepting presence. Macey had assured me that she found my manner "professional" and my thought-provoking questions helpful in an earlier rapport-building phase of work. Proving myself as a reliable and emotionally available provider was crucial to establishing a "holding environment" (Winnicott, 1960). Macey's difficulty being able to rely on her caregivers—both real and symbolic—would end up being a pivotal theme in our work together.

Powerlessness in Shared Space

Macey's mounting sense of powerlessness in response to her family's health difficulties was compounded by an erosion of autonomy in her home. Shortly after her mother-in-law was diagnosed with cancer, her family made the difficult decision to bring both her and Macey's grandmother-in-law into their home so she could have access to quality medical care and be close to family. Without the financial means to secure a separate space, their tight living arrangement quickly became a source of familiar friction over privacy and domestic routines. The beginning phase of our work revolved around providing support for these environmental stressors and attempting to bridge communication difficulties.

Macey had previously seen a therapist for these issues when they were all living together in Eastern Europe shortly after fleeing the war. Her marriage was on the brink of divorce when she convinced her husband they needed to move out into their own space. Returning to this shared arrangement with her in-laws felt like a loss of progress and reopened painful wounds of living with her family in a cramped apartment with communal amenities. As a child, she had to share a room with her two siblings, constantly navigating space and boundaries with them, never feeling like she had anything she could call her own.

The reoccurring displacement since the outbreak of the war and deferment of her lifelong dream of independence started to take a heavy emotional toll on her. These early experiences had instilled a deep desire in Macey to leave her family home and live on her own, a dream she finally realized as an adult when she started a family and moved into an inherited apartment. The resurfacing of these confining conditions forced her to live through the "worst experiences" of her past as "felt emotional realities in the present" (Ecker et al., 2012).

Macey expressed a profound sense of helplessness, feeling like she was in a tunnel with "no end in sight," blocked from coping with the present and imagining a future. Such a collapse and splitting of time is indicative of a traumatic response, leaving one's experiences "sequestered" from the present and without hope for the future (Bryon, 2021). In our earlier sessions, she found relief in my interpretation that her conflicts with her in-laws echoed the dynamics of her suffocating upbringing, where she had felt voiceless and powerless. This insight helped her contextualize her difficulties expressing her needs and moved her toward reclaiming agency (van der Kolk, 2009).

She ended up spending more time away from home with her daughter or helping her husband at his job. Macey sought out small symbols that restored her sense of control amid feelings of powerlessness and a loss of space. She enthusiastically described the wooden spoons and cutting boards that she found at yard sales. For her family, these were just ordinary utensils, but to Macey, they signified a sense of home that she desperately craved, something that she could call "mine." Setting boundaries remained fraught as she often found herself disappointed when her in-laws failed to respect her preferences regarding their care, further withdrawing from them with each transgression. Paradoxically, she bristled when other areas were tidied without her consent, struggling to reconcile her need for order without feeling intruded upon. Through these ambivalences, Macey appeared to be embodying a regressive "'mine' and 'yours' split" when it came to the psychic delineation of her household and the belongings within it (Akhtar, 1995). Though originally used to describe immigrant resistance to cultural integration, this phenomenon can be extended to other facets of life as a result of similar splitting processes that inhibit a shared sense of "us."

With time, Macey was able to create psychological distance between the reliving of her past and her current stressors, enabling a new narrative to emerge. In a particularly insightful moment, Macey shared how she was experiencing the "joy" of a "child" while having the ability to communicate like an "adult." This allowed her to access untapped possibilities and arrive at newfound compromises by relaxing rigid roles and delegating childcare responsibilities to her in-laws. Macey's ability to hold her youthful enthusiasm while embodying a maturing agency signified a growing capacity to inhabit a vital multiplicity of self (Bromberg, 1996).

Loss and Longing for Connection

Therapy opened a symbolic space for Macey where she could heal deeper emotional wounds. She would use our time to give voice to unmet needs and unexpressed yearnings. In one session, she tenderly described caring for a new cutting board by oiling it and protecting it from pungent ingredients. Beyond the implications of control covered in the previous section, this symbolized a nascent expression of affection that was previously inaccessible. Macey's defended state and practical concerns made it difficult for her to let her guard down and make room for spontaneous emotions—like the capacity for play. Even when she expressed warm feelings toward her daughter, she would often include a self-reproach about how she felt she wasn't interested enough in the type of games she enjoyed. Macey started to use the safety of the therapeutic holding environment to experiment with novel ways of being, strengthen inner resources, and process loss (Winnicott, 1960). Revisiting fond memories of collaborating with her husband on their lifestyle blog brought forth adaptive self-states. Macey connected her striving for independence and autonomy to the confidence and enthusiasm she felt when she went off to university. From a fortified sense of self, she started to reconcile unmet emotional needs that stemmed from feeling neglected by her mother, who favored her sister and cherished her younger brother by virtue of him being the only boy. Their forced separation following the invasion further deepened her disconnection from her siblings, as her sister fled to another part of Europe, while her brother remained in Ukraine.

The imbalance of nurturing left her feeling starved for individualized attention and distrustful of her mother. Her longing for affection and wish to feel special would frequently come up in her interpersonal relationships. During my pottery workshop, Macey became frustrated with her husband for making a triangular vase, immediately associating the three sides to represent her and her two in-laws. As a result of this unintended meaning, the vase and their shared experience were symbolically no longer "just for her," evoking both an eroding sense of control and a reminder of her emotional neglect.

Macey shared a memory of her mother impatiently combing her hair and hurting her scalp when she was a child. These early childhood ruptures would lead to the "paradoxical" coupling of what could have been "soothing" with fear in the presence of her caregivers (Liotti, 2011). Macey captured this relational bind in a later session, saying, "When I allow them to come closer, they end up violating my boundaries," and concluding, "I can't accept their help." Her difficulty tolerating closeness intensified the intimacy difficulties in her marriage that were already heightened due to a lack of privacy in their home. Despite craving a closer connection with her husband, Macey shared how she would often tense up when he tried to hug her, unconsciously communicating a need for distance. Her "unresolved fearful affects" would inhibit her from "obtaining" the very "comfort" she sought (Goldner, 2014). She would start to contextualize her conflicting needs as ripples of intergenerational trauma from her maternal side. Macey arrived at the insight that her grandmother's abusive marriage shaped a dysfunctional template of attachment for her mother and aunts, all of them having endured unhappy relationships at one point of their lives (Salberg, 2015). Macey would go on to process how her firsthand experiences of her parents' disordered dynamic left her feeling shaken and overwhelmed. In a vivid retelling of a childhood memory, she described how she hid when her father would come home and yell at her mother for leaving the apartment messy as she struggled to take care of three young kids. Macey retreated to escape the chaos of their fights and was left feeling helpless that she wasn't able to defend her mother. These familiar and paralyzing feelings of powerlessness would resurface throughout her life, coming to a crescendo when the war broke out.

Isolation and the Search for Sanctuary

Macey expressed how traumatizing it was to take refuge in a dusty basement, viscerally recalling the "sensory realities" of the sounds of sirens and explosions amid blackouts. Ten grueling days of sheltering left her with an enduring sense that she would never feel safe there again (Akhtar, 1995). The foreclosed possibility of returning to her homeland made it even more difficult to envision a future as tensions within her marriage intensified. Her husband was feeling increasingly overworked by his demanding cousin and struggling to keep up with rising costs. They had lost precious time to displacement and were now approaching midlife without a sense of direction. He fantasized about starting over in various countries while she worried about how yet another relocation might destabilize her daughter, who had only just made a friend at school. With a heavy sigh, Macey dreaded she would have to "go against her will," bringing back familiar feelings of powerlessness. I found myself deeply resonating with her feelings of helplessness, meeting her glance and looking away, wondering what words could possibly help in the face of such challenging circumstances.

Macey confided how she once hid in a storage closet after work to escape the mounting pressures at home. Though she identified hiking and meditation as ways to decompress from the day and relieve stress, she found it too difficult to advocate for more alone time. Unable to shift out of hyperarousal, moments of solitude often took on a hypervigilant and persecutory feel for her, driven by the fear that she would lose "control" if she ever let her guard down. The war had left her feeling shaken, unable to trust the safety of the present, and left stranded without possibility of returning home (Winnicott, 1958). In my work with other refugees, many reported feeling overwhelmed by such a crushing reality, desperately wishing to come back to the lives and family they left behind. They struggled to overcome the doubt of starting over in a foreign land—it was too daunting to learn an unfamiliar language and integrate into a new way of life. This left them feeling like they were burdening their family members as they further withdrew into themselves and away from the possibility of a future.

Repairing Attachment Through Art and Community

Hearing stories of profound alienation and disillusionment illuminated the devastating impact of the war and the "widespread social change" unfolding in its wake (Bodnar, 2004). As a ceramicist, I was inspired to share the rich tradition of Ukrainian pottery, offering participants a way to internalize and draw strength from a fortifying cultural resource (Drobko, 2024). Macey was skeptical about joining my workshop at first but eventually welcomed the chance to share a new experience with her husband, away from her in-laws.

In an earlier section, we explored how her husband's triangular vase took on unintended associations but enabled us to deepen the work around her family dynamics. This illustrates how participants were able to use the malleable nature of clay to symbolically imbue and derive meaning from their pieces. Many participants imagined the everyday use of their pieces—bowls for fruits, mugs for tea—grounding them to the present. Macey crafted a small cylindrical vase, envisioning that it would hold her daughter's miniature bouquets from their walks together. This created a "tangible vision" that allowed her to begin imagining how she could "bridge the present to the future," planting a metaphorical seed that would one day blossom (Bryon, 2021).

Another participant made a hanging panel with pressed plants from her neighborhood park, symbolizing her deepening integration into a new life. Her unique piece grew from the creative spark of a prior workshop, where she reconnected with her identity as a costume designer. This experience empowered her to start an apprenticeship with a local tattoo artist. I wanted participants to work with a forgiving medium that would give them the freedom to take risks and experiment—something that would feel like play. I fondly recall the laughter and excitement that filled the workshops as they expressed themselves in ways that felt true to them (Lenormand, 2018). A new experience like this can shift one's sense of self and open the door to imagining a life beyond survival and, at times, to rebuilding a sense of "home" through shared connection (Zinfandel & Svensson, 2024). Shortly after the workshop, Macey expressed a desire to celebrate the holidays in a meaningful way, signaling a growing openness to new traditions, marking a shift toward cultural assimilation in contrast to her husband's ongoing ambivalence and resistance (Akhtar, 1995).

Transcending Traditional Boundaries of Care

Macey's step toward greater integration reflected my wishes for the workshop and led me to consider my own multifaceted role. I served not only as her individual therapist but also as her pottery instructor and host—fluidly moving through boundaries as needed, guided less by fixed professional roles than by a flexible, relational stance attuned to the shifting realities of her life (Horowitz, 1998). I wondered whether I was witnessing her process as an attuned clinician or as an artistic mentor, guiding her psychic and creative explorations with a spirit of curiosity and empowerment. The workshop setting had already begun to stretch the boundaries of the traditional therapeutic frame, creating a space where clinical containment, creative expression, and community engagement could come together. This orientation continued to inform my evolving role beyond the therapy room and shaped my involvement in a picnic fundraiser honoring Ukrainian soldiers who had lost their limbs in the war.

Organized in collaboration with a nonprofit specializing in advanced prosthetics for veterans and civilians, the event invited community members to gather, offer support, and contribute their own symbolic gestures through art and performance. I helped with outreach, fundraising, and promotion leading up to the event and then stepped into a facilitative role by leading a collage-making activity that encouraged connection through collective symbolism and creative ritual. The experience invited engagement and healing across intrapsychic, relational, and cultural dimensions within what has been described as a "traumatic field," where individual pain intersects with communal efforts toward repair (Margherita & Tessitore, 2023).

We chose the sunflower, a national symbol of resilience and cultural continuity, as our shared image. As soon as the first piece was placed, children eagerly began arranging shapes and colors, immersed in a sense of play while parents looked on with delight, occasionally stepping in to assist or add pieces of their own. The collage became a natural gathering spot, its own holding environment, inviting the reassembly of what had been scattered into coherence. It also called to mind a technique I'd learned during a lecture on narrative exposure therapy, where individuals place stones and flowers along a physical timeline to mark painful and joyful events (Tissue et al., 2023). In a similar spirit, we saved sunflower petals to give more reserved attendees a chance to contribute a piece of their own story, bringing the collage to life.

Later, I learned a new client had attended the event but felt too shy to introduce herself or join the collage, reflecting the deep sense of withdrawal and alienation she had carried since relocating. I began to wonder what it meant for her to see me in that communal role—how it might shape her understanding of who I was and influence the space between us.

From the outset, our work unfolded beyond the conventional psychoanalytic frame. She had been referred by a local nonprofit offering culinary training for refugees, arriving with a multitude of pressing needs: navigating the shelter system, food insecurity, childcare, work permit delays, and gaps in healthcare. Before we could begin meaningful trauma work, these had to be addressed. I drew on earlier experience in a homeless shelter to help guide her through public assistance systems and partnered with asylum advocates, food networks, and nonprofits on her behalf. Over time, I've come to understand that responding to the evolving realities of our clients is not separate from the work. It is what makes space for what may emerge next.

Resilience During Uncertain Times and Hope for the Future

After the new year, Macey reported a sense of stability in her life and requested to shift to biweekly sessions, feeling that her progress had plateaued. She had reached a place of relative acceptance regarding her in-laws, oscillating between feeling empowered at times and withdrawing at others. We continued at this cadence for two months before she asked to return to weekly meetings, feeling that "too much time had passed by" and signaling a renewed need for support as the impasse with her husband grew and the situation in Ukraine worsened. Macey dreaded the impact that the war would have on her family back home, sharing a disturbing reverie of government authorities going from home to home, collecting the corpses of men, and lowering the draft age—would they survive, would they be the same? (Boss, 1999). Around the same time, the U.S. administration made the decision to revoke the protected status for Ukrainian refugees. Macey was left to navigate an uncertain legal status without a symbolic home to where she could return, saying she felt like "a dog that was taken in, only to be kicked out," echoing the harrowing threat of deportation that so many refugees are facing.

We continued to create new meaning through language, uncovering a theme of "betrayal" in her relationships, rooted in her longing for affection. Macey gave me a knowing smile as she extended this into a broader theme in our work together—"control." A growing sense of mutuality between us made space for moments like these to unfold. In a later session, she expressed how it was hard for her to admit she felt betrayed by me for being less attentive when I was working through a head cold. Providing space for her to voice frustration without the fear of rupture allowed us to move toward greater relatedness (Winnicott, 1949). Being aware of the potential impact of my diminished ability enabled Macey to soften and resonate with my vulnerability (Ehrenberg, 1996). This exchange enabled Macey to connect to her own difficulties with allowing herself to rest, underscoring our shared ethnic background, saying, "We're that kind of people—we push through when the body is telling us to rest." This would be the first time Macey explicitly brought up culture, illustrating its influence within the therapeutic relationship as an active "third presence" (Bodnar, 2004).

The deepening connectivity and expressivity created space for Macey to voice feelings of gratitude and love for her husband. Macey recently expressed that she can't "imagine life without him" and has been encouraged to see the "gleam" in his eyes return when he looks at her. With a restored ability to visualize a hopeful future, Macey reframed their current difficulties as something that would ultimately strengthen their bond. She's been able to "see an end" to the situation with her in-laws when she had previously felt that there was "no end nor edge" to her misery. She notes that she's able to operate from a "resourced" and integrated position more often, giving way for her "kind" personality to shine through, spontaneously singing and making jokes with her family. Our reparative work has solidified her "instinct for self-preservation," leaving her feeling increasingly confident in a time of great uncertainty and instability. Macey is able to hold onto small moments of joy and possibility as she sits in her car, alone with her thoughts, imagining what it would be like to live "somewhere else," in touch with a sense of "freedom."

Toward a Psychoanalysis Without Borders

Fundamentally, the RSP is an applied psychoanalytic approach to healing social trauma. The program recognizes that psychic suffering is never isolated from historical, political, or communal realities. By situating clinical work within a matrix of social action, RSP operationalizes an expanded psychoanalytic framework, one attuned to both inner psychic states and the external conditions of displacement and oppression.

Looking ahead, RSP aims to deepen its integration within PPSC and further anchor the institute's commitment to social repair. The success of this initiative has revealed significant potential to expand the scope and application of psychoanalytic work to social causes. It has also catalyzed a number of interconnected initiatives at PPSC, positioning applied psychoanalysis as an exciting new frontier. In all of this, RSP seeks not merely to stabilize the lives of those affected by trauma, exile, and war but to support the recovery of their full humanity and, in doing so, to reimagine psychoanalysis as a practice of collective healing without borders.

References

Ainslie, R. (2017). Immigration, psychic dislocation, and the re-creation of community. *Psychoanalytic Review*, *104*(6), 695–706. https://doi.org/10.1521/prev.2017.104.6.695

Akhtar, S. (1995). A third individuation: Immigration, identity, and the psychoanalytic process. *Journal of the American Psychoanalytic Association*, *43*, 1051–1084. https://doi.org/10.1177/000306519504300406

Alayarian, A. (2019). Trauma, resilience and healthy and unhealthy forms of dissociation. *Journal of Analytical Psychology*, *64*(4), 587–606. https://doi.org/10.1111/1468-5922.12522

Altman, N. (1993). Psychoanalysis and the urban poor. *Psychoanalytic Dialogues*, *3*(1), 29–49. https://doi.org/10.1080/10481889309538958

Bodnar, S. (2004). Remember where you come from: Dissociative process in multicultural individuals. *Psychoanalytic Dialogues*, *14*(5), 581–603. https://doi.org/10.1080/10481880409353128

Boss, P. (1999). *Ambiguous loss: Learning to live with unresolved grief*. Harvard University Press. https://doi.org/10.2307/j.ctvjhzrh4

Boulanger, G. (2008). Witnesses to reality: Working psychodynamically with survivors of terror. *Psychoanalytic Dialogues*, *18*(5), 638–657. https://doi.org/10.1080/10481880802297673

Boulanger, G., & Rosenberg, L. M. (2023). Introduction to second special issue: Psychodynamic interventions in community mental health: We have come full circle! *International Journal of Applied Psychoanalytic Studies*, *20*(4), 537–539. https://doi.org/10.1002/aps.1851

Bromberg, P. M. (1996). Standing in the spaces: The multiplicity of self and the psychoanalytic relationship. *Contemporary Psychoanalysis*, *32*(4), 509–535. https://doi.org/10.1080/00107530.1996.10746334

Bryon, D. (2021). Processing trauma in psychoanalysis in "real" time and in dreams: The convergence of past, present and future during COVID-19. *Journal of Analytical Psychology*, *66*(3), 399–410. https://doi.org/10.1111/1468-5922.12695

Drobko, A. (2024). *Ceramics/Кераміка [Ukrainian ceramics]*. University of Kansas, Center for Russian, East European & Eurasian Studies. https://crees.ku.edu/ukrainian-ceramics

Ecker, B., Ticic, R., & Hulley, L. (2012). *Unlocking the emotional brain: Eliminating symptoms at their roots using memory reconsolidation*. (1st ed.). Routledge. https://doi.org/10.4324/9780203804377

Ehrenberg, D. B. (1996). On the analyst's emotional availability and vulnerability. *Contemporary Psychoanalysis*, *32*(2), 275–286. https://doi.org/10.1080/00107530.1996.10746953

Fisher, J. (2015). *Healing the fragmented selves of trauma survivors: Overcoming internal self-alienation*. Routledge. https://doi.org/10.4324/9781315886169

Freud, S. (1990). *The question of lay analysis* (J. Strachey, Trans. & Ed.). W. W. Norton & Company. (Original work published 1926)

Goldner, V. (2014). Romantic bonds, binds, and ruptures: Couples on the brink. *Psychoanalytic Dialogues, 24*(4), 402–418. https://doi.org/10.1080/10481885.2014.932209

Hollander, N. C. (2010). *Uprooted minds: Surviving the politics of terror in the Americas*. Routledge.

Holmes, D. E., Hart, A. H., Powell, D. R., Stoute, B. J., Chodorow, N. J., Davids, M. F., Dennis, E., Glover, W., González, F. J., Hamer, F. M., Javier, R. A., Katz, M., Leary, K. R., Maree, R. D., Méndez, T., Moskowitz, M., Moss, D., Tummala-Narra, P., Ueng-McHale, J., Vaughans, K. C., … McNamara, S. (Ed.) (2024). In pursuit of racial equality in American psychoanalysis: Findings and recommendations from the Holmes Commission. *Journal of the American Psychoanalytic Association, 72*(3), 407–552. https://doi.org/10.1177/00030651241253623

Horowitz, J. (1998). Contemporary psychoanalysis and social work theory. *Clinical Social Work Journal, 26*(4), 369–383. https://doi.org/10.1023/A:1022873920417

Jacoby, R. (1983). *The repression of psychoanalysis: Otto Fenichel and the political Freudians*. Basic Books.

Kane, B. S. (2005). Transforming trauma into tragedy: Oedipus/Israel and the psychoanalyst as messenger. *Psychoanalytic Review, 92*, 929–956. https://doi.org/10.1521/prev.2005.92.6.929

Kirsner, D. (2000). *Unfree associations: Inside psychoanalytic institutes*. Jason Aronson.

Klein, M. (1946). Notes on some schizoid mechanisms. *International Journal of Psychoanalysis, 27*, 99–110. https://psycnet.apa.org/record/1948-02558-001

Koh, E., & Twemlow, S. W. (2018). Towards a psychoanalytic concept of community (IV): The well-functioning community. *International Journal of Applied Psychoanalytic Studies, 15*, 5–15. https://doi.org/10.1002/aps.1527

Kohut, H. (2010). On empathy: Heinz Kohut (Original work published 1981). *International Journal of Psychoanalytic Self Psychology, 5*(2), 122–131. https://psycnet.apa.org/record/2010-07556-002

Layton, L. (2006). Attacks on linking: The unconscious pull to dissociate individuals from their social context. In L. Layton, N. C. Hollander, & S. Gutwill (Eds.), *Psychoanalysis, class and politics: Encounters in the clinical setting* (pp. 107–117). Routledge.

Lenormand, S. (2018). Winnicott's theory of playing: A reconsideration. *The International Journal of Psychoanalysis, 99*(1), 82–102. https://doi.org/10.1080/00207578.2017.1399068

Liotti, G. (2011). Attachment disorganization and the controlling strategies: An illustration of the contributions of attachment theory to developmental psychopathology and to psychotherapy integration. *Journal of Psychotherapy Integration, 21*(3), 232–252. https://doi.org/10.1037/a0025422

Luci, M. (2020). Displacement as trauma and trauma as displacement in the experience of refugees. *Journal of Analytical Psychology*, *65*(2), 260–280. https://doi.org/10.1111/1468-5922.12590

Margherita, G., & Tessitore, F. (2023). Facing the traumatic field in the clinical and social work with forced migrants through a psychodynamic perspective: From "refugee trauma" to the clinic of social links. *Clinical Social Work Journal*, *51*(4), 379–388. https://doi.org/10.1007/s10615-023-00894-y

Minozzo, A., & Soreanu, R. (2024). On the mental health commons: Brazilian free psychoanalytic clinics and an ethics of togetherness. *Critical Times*, *7*(3), 423–447. https://doi.org/10.1215/26410478-11394879

Ogden, P., Pain, C., & Fisher, J. (2006). A sensorimotor approach to the treatment of trauma and dissociation. *Psychiatric Clinics of North America*, *29*(1), 263–279. https://doi.org/10.1016/j.psc.2005.10.012

Onofrio, G. B., & Kitroser, N. (2021). Psychodynamic psychiatry in Argentina at a crossroads. *Psychodynamic Psychiatry*, *49*(3), 379–383. https://doi.org/10.1521/pdps.2021.49.3.379

Orange, D. M. (2016). *The ethical turn in psychoanalysis: Critical perspectives on the humanities and the social sciences*. Routledge.

Oury, J. (2024). Institutional psychotherapy: From Saint-Alban to La Borde. In M. Miguel & E. Vogman (Eds.), *Psychotherapy and materialism: Essays* (pp. 89–119). *Cultural Inquiry*, 31. ICI Berlin Press. https://doi.org/10.37050/ci-31_04

Rose, G. J. (1990). From ego-defense to reality enhancement: Updating the analytic perspective on art. *The American Imago*, *47*(1), 69–79. http://www.jstor.org/stable/26303966

Saakvitne, K. W. (2002). Shared trauma: The therapist's increased vulnerability. *Psychoanalytic Dialogues*, *12*(3), 443–449. https://doi.org/10.1080/10481881209348678

Salberg, J. (2015). The Texture of traumatic attachment: Presence and ghostly absence in trans-generational transmissions. *The Psychoanalytic Quarterly*, *84*(1), 21–46. https://doi.org/10.1002/j.2167-4086.2015.00002.x

Statista. (2025, April 17). *Ukrainian refugees worldwide 2025*. https://www.statista.com/statistics/1413699/ukrainian-refugees-worldwide/

Stern, D. B. (1983). Unformulated experience: From familiar chaos to creative disorder. *Contemporary Psychoanalysis*, *19*(1), 71–99. https://doi.org/10.1080/00107530.1983.10746593

Stern, D. B. (2017). Unformulated experience, dissociation, and nachträglichkeit. *The Journal of Analytic Psychology*, *62*(4), 501–525. https://doi.org/10.1111/1468-5922.12334

Tissue, A., Specker, P., Hoffman, J., Uppal, S., Cloitre, M., Neuner, F., O'Donnell, M., & Nickerson, A. (2023). Skills training in affective and interpersonal regulation for refugees integrated with narrative exposure therapy: A case study on the treatment of PTSD and emotion dysregulation for refugees and asylum-seekers. *Clinical Case Studies*, *22*(3), 285–306. https://doi.org/10.1177/15346501221133315

van der Kolk, B. A. (1994). The body keeps the score: Memory and the evolving psychobiology of post-traumatic stress. *Harvard Review of Psychiatry, 1*(5), 253–265. https://doi.org/10.3109/10673229409017088

van der Kolk, B. A. (2002). Posttraumatic therapy in the age of neuroscience. *Psychoanalytic Dialogues, 12*(3), 381–392. https://doi.org/10.1080/10481881209348674

van der Kolk, B. A. (2009). *The body keeps the score: Brain, mind, and body in the healing of trauma*. Viking.

Winnicott, D. W. (1949). Hate in the counter-transference. *International Journal of Psychoanalysis, 30*, 69–74. https://psycnet.apa.org/record/1950-06381-001

Winnicott, D. W. (1958). The capacity to be alone. *International Journal of Psychoanalysis, 39*, 416–420. https://psycnet.apa.org/record/1960-02846-001

Winnicott, D. W. (1960). The theory of the parent-infant relationship. *International Journal of Psychoanalysis, 41*, 585–595. https://pep-web.org/browse/document/IJP.041.0585A

Winograd, B. (Director). (2014). *Black psychoanalysts speak* [Documentary film]. PEP Video Grants.

Zaleski, K. L., Johnson, D. K., & Klein, J. T. (2016). Grounding Judith Herman's trauma theory within interpersonal neuroscience and evidence-based practice modalities for trauma treatment. *Smith College Studies In Social Work, 86*(4), 377–393. https://doi.org/10.1080/00377317.2016.1222110

Zinfandel, S., & Svensson, M. (2024). Fostering trust – A qualitative outcome study of psychodynamic group and individual psychotherapy for refugees with PTSD. *European Journal of Psychotraumatology, 15*(1). https://doi.org/10.1080/20008066.2024.2413736

Chapter 2

From Destruction to Growth

Multimodal Psychoanalytic Aid for War-Traumatized Chechen Children*

Nina Cerfolio

Let's start with hope. After providing medical and psychological care in New York to Chechen children who were victims of the Second Chechen War, our humanitarian team brought them to a festive party at the Lighthouse Guild party for blind children. As the Chechen children and I entered the space decorated with balloons and food-filled tables, they suddenly morphed into familiar, giddy children who could squeal at opening Christmas stockings. Their vibrant smiles were contagious. Momentarily suspended from their enveloping grief, the Chechens had an astonishing innate social ease that erupted in meeting other disabled children and enjoying the plentiful and varied food that was served. Their joyful spontaneity released the confines of my professional harness as a physician, medical advocate, and coordinator, allowing me to reveal myself as their playful companion. Wearing my favorite blue dress, I transformed into an unburdened partier. Displaying a pure sense of gratitude, the children eased into a flowing reciprocity of genuine connection and concern. I proudly introduced them to the other children, and despite the language barrier, I felt closely bonded to them. After the party, I ensured that they had transportation to where we had provided housing for them during their stay in New York City. They, in turn, showed their protective regard for my safety by inquiring how

* Note. Portions of this chapter expand on material previously published in the following works:
From *Multimodal psychoanalytically informed aid work with children traumatized by the Chechen War*, by N. Cerfolio, 2009, Guilford Press. Copyright 2009 by Guilford Press. Reproduced by permission of Guilford Press.
From *Psychoanalytic and spiritual perspectives on terrorism: Desire for destruction* (1st ed.), by N. Cerfolio, 2023, Routledge. Copyright 2023 by Routledge. Reproduced by permission of Taylor & Francis Group.

DOI: 10.4324/9781003658382-3

I was getting home after the party. Becoming part of my metaphorical family, the Chechens had forever entered my heart (Cerfolio, 2023).

We need to remember the Chechens' struggle for independence from Russia dating back to 1785, when Catherine the Great's forces encountered Chechen mountain resistance fighters. History that is forgotten often repeats itself. There are global consequences when the world turns a blind eye to Putin's unopposed 20 years of waging wars in Chechnya beginning in 1994, Georgia in 2008, Crimea in 2014, and Syria in 2015. The historical lack of global resistance concerning this Russian aggression emboldened an alarming normalization of Putin to continue with his tyrannical waging of wars and murdering of innocent civilians in Ukraine (Cerfolio, 2023).

Russia is not alone in waging wars, as this is emblematic and a part of American history and mythology. In modern thought, we have married the relentlessly ubiquitous presence of evil, which is understood by the Shakespearean utterance, "The fault, dear Brutus, is not in the stars, But in ourselves." How do we come to terms with the realization of our own unconscious motivations that create war and destroy lives? How do we understand evil and the dynamics of war, which involves killing and dying out of love of country? How do we bear witness to the Ukrainians' suffering and remain attuned to finding ways to support the challenges of Russian acts of terror that the Ukrainian people are enduring?

Similar to Hitler's desire to purify and unify Germany, Putin's justification of his war in Ukraine is the creation of a highly desired "sacred" empire based on Christian fascism and fundamentalism, which the Orthodox Church fully supports (Lifton, 2022). This Christian fascism centers on a unified, godly Russian empire achieved by Peter the Great that is pure in its virtue and absolute in its justified demands. The Russian leader said that one of the goals of the offensive was to "denazify" Ukraine, part of a long-running effort by Putin to delegitimize Ukrainian nationalism and sell the incursion to his constituency at home. The rhetoric around fighting fascism resonates deeply in Russia, which made tremendous sacrifices battling Nazi Germany in World War II. Critics say that Putin is exploiting the trauma of that war and twisting history for his own interests.

A deeper trigger for Russia's invasion may not have been "self-purification" but Putin's refusal to admit that neighboring Ukraine had become a flourishing democracy. The contrast of Ukrainian democratic success would have been intolerable for Putin and may be one reason why he is trying to erase Ukraine. Putin was never going to let a Slavic Ukraine become a successful free-market democracy in the European Union next door to his stagnating Slavic Russian kleptocracy.

In the past, the world became inured to the brutality inflicted by Putin in the Russian wars in Chechnya, Syria, and Georgia. In sharp contrast, there has been an incredible outpouring of international aid in response to Putin's "special military operation" in Ukraine. This support was inspired in part by the brave resistance of the Ukrainian people, but also because the West may more readily identify with Ukrainians, who, as Slavic people, are perceived to share certain racial and cultural traits with some European and North American people. Perhaps those in power's identification with the Ukrainian people, as opposed to the Chechen Muslims, allows the world to more readily recognize their suffering, open its heart, and offer help.

While doing firsthand humanitarian aid work during the Second Chechen War, I personally witnessed the sequelae of the world's laxness in not protesting Russia's destructive war crimes against Chechens. Similarly, Putin specializes in weaponizing refugees in an attempt to create resentment and destabilization of neighboring republics and countries. America seemed to tolerate Putin's waging war in Asia, in part, echoing 19th-century colonization and to skip past the specter of nuclear devastation. But then the world suddenly woke up and showed unity in protesting Putin's invasion of Ukraine. Although many countries have not followed through with direct actions, the global resolve of citizenry remains unflinching and immovable.

When one cannot contain feelings like rage, vengeance, and envy, the Other may become the repository of these projected unwanted, disowned feelings. Despite decades of Putin's waging war and killing innocent Muslim civilians, our country's lack of response revealed a process of "othering" Muslim suffering. When we inflict wars on our brothers and sisters, we ignore the fact that human experience is composed of multiplicity. As the pursuit of virtue becomes a scarce commodity, it further tatters our sense of community and spiritual connectedness (Cerfolio, 2016). Othering creates a divisiveness that falsely insists that we are superior and that it is acceptable to humiliate and exploit those we do not identify with. This primitive tribalism foments much of the conflict in the world. Only by developing capacities to bear witness to the suffering of all, especially those from marginalized races and cultures, do we begin to reconnect severed social links and heal our world with the recognition of the unity of our planet (Davoine & Gaudillière, 2004).

A Paradigm for Care: Multimodal Psychoanalytic Aid with Children Traumatized by the Second Chechen War

This has all been a preamble for your understanding of my sentiments that galvanized me to go into the Second Chechen War to help—not a popular choice in my family. To address the suffering, in August of 2005, I visited Chechnya with a colleague to provide medical care to those stranded in Grozny and the Chechen refugees in Ingushetia. We also started a disabled running club chapter in New York to help those who became amputees as a result of the war and to bring disabled Chechen children to New York for further medical treatment (Cerfolio, 2009). Although our team helped many Chechens—both refugees living in neighboring Ingushetia and those trapped in war-torn Grozny received medical and psychological care—I will focus primarily on our efforts with providing care to two Chechen children we met in Grozny and were able to bring to New York for continued care. Being a volunteer in this running club, including serving on the Board of Advisors, the board of the Track Club for Disabled Iraqi War Veterans, and as an athlete due to a post-lenticular cataract which contributed to legal blindness in my right eye, I have experienced firsthand the empowerment of running to overcome life's obstacles and improve mental health. As a result of our visit, 300 disabled Chechen children ran a 5-kilometer race in Ingushetia on September 11, 2005. It marked the first time a Muslim republic banded together officially to run against terrorism. In June 2007, after two years of emails and telephone calls, and six failures with their exit visas, the children arrived for their six-week stay in New York. Thanks to the support of several nonprofit organizations, the children received prosthetics and medical care, and their transportation, airfare, and room and board were completely funded. The medical team consisted of two rehabilitation physicians, a medical internist, a prosthetist, a translator, and me, a psychoanalytic psychiatrist.

It is important to note that a multimodal psychoanalytic framework—including but not restricted to those represented by the Freudian, interpersonal, and relational orientations—was essential to work through countertransference, remain present, and provide medical care to these traumatized Chechen children. With the translator, I saw the children individually and as a group five days a week; I also ran with each of the children biweekly in scheduled workouts in Central Park and saw them at other social and athletic functions. The medical team met weekly to define psychological and medical treatment guidelines for each child and to set up daily activities, coordinate care, and identify and deal with the children's individual coping difficulties experienced by transitioning from a war-torn environment to a place to rebuild their resilience.

In the planning stages of our effort, our medical goal had been to bring back children with below-the-knee amputations (BKA), as we determined that BKA could be medically addressed within the limits of both the six-week stay in New York and the limited follow-up medical resources available in Chechnya. Despite our recommendations, and due to understandable circumstances beyond our control, two children were brought who had extensive injuries and who were limited in their recovery by both the practical and medical considerations of their six-week stay.

In an effort to contribute to the understanding of the psychological impact of war on children, we focused on Chechnya, since the Chechen War has been one of the most dangerous, least reported, and least understood. There is a tremendous need for medically and psychoanalytically trained aid workers in this area. The risk of nonintervention is that the next generation of Chechens will feel a deepening isolation as they struggle alone with the emotional and physical toll the war brought. By this point in their history, the Chechen sense of vulnerability has increased, as their struggle has been largely ignored internationally; much of the violence that occurred in Chechnya was not reported by the world press due in part to the political agenda of the United States. The United States was eager to link the Chechens' fight against militant separatists in the North Caucasus with the international struggle against terror (Goldfarb & Litvinenko, 2007). Consequently, the Chechens' sense of hopelessness has left them vulnerable to the lure of terrorism as a means to create awareness of their struggle for survival (Cerfolio,

2020a, 2020b, 2020c, 2024). It was vitally important that other options be presented, and our team found that by grounding our work in the Chechen culture and engaging with individuals—listening and attending to their experience—we developed a deeper understanding of their needs. Reaching out to them, the medical team began to attend to their emotional, mental, and physical needs to chip away at the hopelessness and despair that is often a breeding ground for extremist response and terrorism. We hoped that this important therapeutic intervention presented a different paradigm that would take seed in these Chechen children's lives to help them envision the possibility of a more peaceful and hopeful future and put them on a path of healing.

It was difficult to predict how survivors would respond to the re-education and training required for them to work through potentially unrealistic expectations and accept the limitations of their medical situation. Our team needed to set realistic limits and boundaries, tolerate the child's (and in the second case, the parent's) potential anger without retaliation, and avoid making unrealistic promises. Each child's situation needed constant reevaluation to ensure that we clearly defined the medical limits of recovery and dealt with the child's emotional response. With this approach, feelings of betrayal, which are common countertransference enactments with trauma survivors, were minimized and both the child and our team had a more rewarding experience.

Review of Literature

When working with traumatized individuals, it is essential to be familiar with the multiple manifestations of the traumatic event on both the child's and analyst's psyche. A key issue in working with traumatized individuals is that traumatic memories are processed differently in the brain than normal memories. Rather than being integrated through the mediation of the hippocampus and prefrontal cortex, traumatic memories are short-circuited and stored as somatic sensations and visual images in the amygdala (Boulanger, 2005). Consequently, traumatic memory can initially only be expressed nonverbally. Memory for trauma has its own language, and verbalization is not the primary one. Moreover, work with survivor testimonies demonstrates that unconscious and repressed memory traces are not preserved intact but are subject to complex modifications (Krystal, 2004).

Among the unique attributes of working with a traumatized individual is his or her altered sense of time. Trauma seems to fragment the individual's experience of continuous time. The past seems to coexist with the present, and trauma is experienced as a current event, but it is not always consciously accessible. Memories of trauma are painful to remember as well as hard to forget. They may be remembered, forgotten, and then remembered over again (Grand, 1995; Heim & Nemeroff, 2001; Hoffman, 2004; Nemeroff, 2004; Person & Klar, 1994; Rothe, 2008; Vinar, 2003). One of the major reverberations that results from these issues is that survivors of massive human-made psychic trauma frequently experience deficits in symbolic functioning affecting their capacity to think productively (Bromberg, 2000; Laub & Auerhahn, 1989, 1993; Prince, 1998).

In the therapeutic milieu, affect dysregulation is a familiar problem for the analytic dyad when the patient is a victim of trauma (Bromberg, 2000). The return of the traumatic memories with associated intense affect is understood as the product of dissociated affect and knowledge of the traumatic material, and it creates profound implications for patient, analyst, and the analytic relationship. Memory for trauma can come as an enactment rather than through the prefrontal lobe, as in normal memory. The centrality of enactment of trauma in the clinical situation is well-recognized (Boulanger, 2005; Bromberg, 2000; Prince, 1998). Indeed, the contribution of psychoanalysis to the human understanding of trauma may well be understood best through enactments. Affect dysregulation tests the ability of the analyst to withstand the patient's affective storms; in doing so, the analyst can reaffirm the patient's sense that one can survive those storms, thereby serving as a role model for the patient to withstand his or her own affect.

As a way of understanding the clinical material that follows, it is essential to be familiar with the Chechen historical and cultural background. A 6,000-square-mile corner of the northern Caucasus, Chechnya is one of seven ethnic republics within the Russian Federation. The seven republics' history is closely intertwined; at the time of our visit, half of Chechnya's population was estimated to be living in refugee camps in Ingushetia, a neighboring republic. This placed a tremendous strain on the tiny republic and, in turn, adversely affected the Chechen–Ingush relationship.

Chechnya has struggled for centuries under Russian domination, and its declaration of independence in 1991 led to the most recent war. One of the main cultural differences responsible for the ongoing conflict is religion. Instead of the Russian Orthodox religion practiced in much of Russia, the majority of Chechens are Sunni Muslims.

When we visited in 2005, the Consolidated Appeals Processes[1] estimated that the majority of the people living in Chechnya could not leave, and more than 2,000 children under the age of three would die each year as a result of inadequate medical care. Although the numbers were not definitely known, it is estimated that more than 30,000 Chechen children were injured or killed because of the war or the land mines spread throughout the country. They experienced acts of terrorism, kidnappings, and violence on a daily basis, which further isolated them from the rest of the world. In addition to this horror, UNICEF reported that from 1994 up to 2008, 25,000 children in Chechnya lost one or both parents (Seierstad, 2008). The special emotional bond known to people subjected to genocide, that "never again" sentiment that reduces the whole world to the struggle for survival, has served to unify the Chechens over many generations (Politkovskaya, 2003).

Although Russia has a history of endured persecutions, famines, gulag camps, torture, and organized state murder for most of the 20th century, the notion of trauma is not easy to apply to its people. Historian Catherine Merridale observes with some wonder that the Russians strongly deny any notion of deep psychic damage originating from these events (Merridale, 2001). Post-traumatic stress disorder (PTSD) is not a diagnosis that they seek, and not a label worn with pride. Two considerations may explain this attitude: the fact that mental distress, far from leading to compensation, has been stigmatized in post-Soviet Russia, and that in their earlier history there was no viable alternative than for the people to not discuss some of the things that troubled them.

Other cultural considerations may also play a role in the general Russian denial of trauma among those affected by it. In the Russian milieu, the individual mind is not viewed as the center of every human world. Words like "collectivism" and "social effort" come up when former Soviet citizens attempt to explain why Stalin's Russia did not collapse under its burden of despair. It seems as if our Western concept of individuality and the self strikes the Russian sensibility as amusing.

Moreover, in Russian culture, the losses and persecutions may be tolerated due to a cultural history of suffering, so it is accepted as an honorable position that is part of the human condition. Rather than admit the level of suffering, though, there is a tradition in Russian culture to hide trauma and loss with fabricated versions of the truth. The Russian parent believes that if they deny that something bad has happened and prevent themself from showing the feelings they have about this trauma, they will save and spare their child the pain of these feelings (Konkov, 2001).

Similar cultural values were evident to me in 2005 during our visit to Grozny where, despite block after block being a ravaged wasteland scarred with the detritus of ferocious bombings, the Chechens walked the streets prideful of what little they had, dressed as if they were going to their offices. It was in this hollowed-out place that 90,000–190,000 Chechens made their home. It was hard to imagine Grozny as a once-bustling modern city of education and culture; it became clearer that the attempts to erase the Chechen population from global consciousness had resulted in a cultural anxiety of intense pride and the need to appear "whole." This concrete and intrapsychic perception of wholeness was especially important to the sense of Chechen national pride.

Wars, in general, promote a regression from the depressive position and mobilization of the paranoid-schizoid mechanisms of splitting and projection, as defined by Melanie Klein (1975); there is also a regression to part-object relationships, which exclude empathy, compassion, and concern particularly for out-groups. The situation for the Chechens is compounded by other factors as well. In the case of the Chechen survivors, the processes of symbolization and sublimation were shattered by the enforced regression in refugee camps to the concreteness and realness of biological need. In addition, the Russian government's lack of acknowledgment of the whereabouts of Chechens who were kidnapped and disappeared has fostered a paranoid-schizoid position among the Chechen populace. Because of the lack of knowledge of how a loved one died and the lack of a body, it is more difficult to validate the death and mourn the loss and thereby achieve the depressive position. There is a sense of inner emptiness, which children experience during arrested mourning, when they feel they have been deceived about the death of their parents or grandparent. Survivor guilt is often at the core of arrested mourning for these children (Valent, 1998).

An Example of How a Traumatic Life-Metaphor Was Resolved at an Embodied, Rather Than an Exclusively Verbal, Level

Ali's story illustrates how effective aid work can be when both medical and psychological conditions are met. Ali was an unusually resilient 17-year-old male with a left BKA resulting from injuries caused by a landmine explosion when he was eight. It was medically recommended he come for treatment in New York, where he received a new prosthetic for his BKA. Ali was an architecture student, and, since his father was killed during the war when he was 6, he lived with his mother. Appearing malnourished, Ali had soulful brown eyes beyond his years, a mass of dark curls, and a gentle expression; he was a handsome, engaging, and sensitive young man. He possessed a sense of humor and maturity well beyond his age. We developed an abiding relationship that was cemented when, functioning as his guide, I ran with Ali in the Hope and Possibility race in Central Park. Despite his exposure to oppression, starvation, and other conditions of living in a war zone that were in sharp contrast to the materialistic abundance of the West, Ali flourished in New York. He was sociable and had an amazing inner flexibility and resilience. Ali was somehow able to transform the legacy of his trauma while in New York and take in what was offered.

In *Child Therapy in the Great Outdoors* (2004), Sebastiano Santostefano puts forth that for a child, traumatic life-metaphors may be resolved at an embodied, rather than an exclusively verbal, level. More specifically, they may be resolved as they are enacted between child and therapist in the outdoors. By running together in Central Park, relational psychoanalysts would argue, an understanding can be conveyed to a patient or analyst through nonverbal actions. For example, Ali seemed apprehensive of descending hills, and each time we approached a decline in our five-mile loop in Central Park, we would slow down almost to a halt, his discomfort manifested by his facial and body movements. Even though Ali did not express his feelings verbally, seeing his physical expression of agitation led me to believe he was re-experiencing a previous trauma, possibly the landmine accident itself, during which he fell sideways down a ravine. Perhaps, by creating more space to experience his understandable distress in the presence of a living-witness—my presence—Ali was better able each time to process his painful emotions when coming upon a descent and become more likely to construct an embodied solution to the meaning of this fear. Eventually, Ali was able to create a new way of descending with his two-arm crutches—he would swing them alternatively outward so that he descended the hill with his body being thrown in a zigzag motion. In this manner, his body would be thrown in the opposite direction of his arm crutch, and he would catch his body weight with the other crutch. As Ali internalized the solutions he enacted with me, his embodied self was revised and a new embodied self emerged. This new self enabled Ali to interact with human and nonhuman environments in ways that then promoted his further development. Ultimately, he was able to descend more confidently and with a newfound freedom. My embodied self was also revised as I internalized enactments experienced during our exercise regimen together, and I relied on this revised matrix of embodied metaphors to help my other patients by being able to be more present with them as they transformed fear into action. Taking our therapy to a revised matrix of an embodied life-metaphor, we relied on our non-verbal vocabulary to move from a relational crisis to an enacted solution.

By coming to New York, Ali was able to build upon the emotional and physical recovery that he had already started in his homeland, exemplifying the idea that "experiences wherein child survivors learn to validate their identities without shame, to retrieve memories, and to find their life-purpose have been found to be helpful" (Valent, 1998). For instance, he recalled having lost what had brought him joy—Grozny's cultural and architectural treasures—describing how the national museum was bombed after Russian forces looted what they deemed worthy, such as European paintings, while Chechen art was blown to pieces. While in New York, Ali described and was able to further mourn the loss of buildings built in the 12th century that were leveled to the ground. Ali integrated his life by emotionally confronting his memories of what he had survived, without shame, and when he returned, he continued pursuing his dreams of becoming an architect to rebuild war-torn Grozny.

Ali seemed to have had a fortunate developmental history that facilitated more mature defenses and a flexible coping style that allowed him to deal with the extraordinary atrocities he had experienced. As though he was doggedly unwilling to wean, a noted idiosyncrasy of Ali was his shunning of all liquids at meals except for his notable dedication to milk with dinner. Using humor as a mature defense, Ali was able to take in what we offered and give of himself to others. Not only did he express overwhelming gratitude for what was provided, but he was empathic as well.

In Kleinian terms, Ali's ability to recognize his own aggression (expressed through empathic humor) and to experience and express mourning for his many losses was characteristic of the depressive position. Ali's gratitude was closely bound up with his ability to be generous and expansive. His good internal object allowed him an inner wealth to draw upon in a foreign environment. Being able to express his sadness and mourn his many losses, Ali was at a more highly integrated level of recovery. Auerhahn and Laub (1994) state that the survivors of atrocities, at best, oscillate between images of annihilation and nurturance. Ali was impressively able to hold onto the brutal imagery of his past atrocities but still maintain a nurturing connection to his caregivers, who offered some hope.

With the analytic process depending on the symbolic representation of experience, Ali and I shared the function of bearing witness to the war crimes that he survived. The therapeutic position during witnessing is not that of holder but that of accompanier, the one who stands by. While holding assumes merging, witnessing a painful internal truth requires the assumption of otherness. "In witnessing, we acknowledge the genuineness of what we grasp of the other, while at the same time acknowledging that we can never fully know or grasp what is essential in our patient's otherness" (Ullman, 2006). Ultimately, witnessing and listening to Ali's story may have encouraged a way of further restoring his resilient sense of dignity and further undermining the split between self and enemy.

The Analyst's Role as Witness: How "Being with" Facilitates Change in Trauma-Impacted Parents

This case illustrates the challenges involved in providing medical care for the child of a traumatized parent and the need to be multimodal psychoanalytically informed in withstanding the parent's affective storms, reshaping his trauma experience as an object of memory, and working through the enactments that accompany them. Even when the medical condition was suboptimal, the parent was still able to work through his maelstroms of anger toward further acceptance and gratitude.

Anzor was a 53-year-old married man, father to five children, and caretaker of Malika, his disabled, nonambulatory daughter. He had served in the Russian army and was single-mindedly directed in his mission to help his daughter. While I was in Grozny in 2005, Anzor was charming. He had shown me an earlier photo of Malika, which was proudly displayed on his desk. The photo revealed a plump, well-developed, groomed, rosy-cheeked neonate, but it served as an anodyne disguise for her horrendous medical history. During the 2001 Russian bombing of Grozny, which killed over 100,000 civilian Chechens, Malika was delivered in an underground shelter. Her delivery was complicated by premature rupture of membranes and anoxic encephalopathy. Once her medical charts were translated, Malika's medical diagnosis was unclear since her Chechen medical work-up had been limited. We expressed our concern to her father at that time that we might not be able to significantly improve her medical status. Despite our medical recommendations against it, Anzor brought his now seven-year-old disabled daughter to New York.

When I first met Malika, she was being carried by her father. Malika was unable to walk, spoke only a few words of Chechen, and was incontinent of stool. She did not attend school and was carried, fed, and changed by her father. Tears filled my eyes as I was touched by the loving tenderness and devotion of this father for his disabled daughter. He tied Malika's disabilities to the struggle of his country, saying that for 300 years, they were fighting for freedom and independence, but now they're fighting to survive.

While in New York City, Malika received a diagnosis of spastic cerebral palsy (CP). Her temperament was affable, sweet, and loving; she seemed alert, intelligent, and sensitive to her surroundings. Over the six weeks, Malika received a wheelchair and extensive medical care and rehabilitation. However, she would still need ongoing and intensive speech, cognitive, and physical therapy.

Despite his sophistication in negotiating systems, Anzor's lack of medical knowledge and wish for his daughter to be healthy contributed to his having magical expectations for his daughter's cure. This was, in part, exacerbated by his idealized belief that America is "the land of freedom with the promise that everything is possible." After his daughter's initial medical visit, Anzor was visibly upset and angry. Despite struggling to hold back my tears as I felt responsible both for bringing them to New York and for his suffering, I struggled to approach him more assertively in order to try to explain the limited positive outcomes we could expect. He was convinced that his daughter needed "brain surgery by an American doctor" in order to reverse the damage caused during her traumatic birth. As this was not a reasonable outcome for Malika's condition, I tried to explain that the damage was permanent and that only a slow and constant rehabilitation could incrementally affect her development.

Feeling deflated and powerless, Anzor expressed frustration toward the doctors caring for his daughter and did not want to be compliant with follow-up visits. Initially, Anzor was unable to overcome his feelings of hopelessness and felt resentment. He asked me if the physician, a top ranked and world renowned New York City physiatrist, who was treating his daughter was "a real doctor?" At one point, he expressed his belief that his daughter's medical problems resulted from poisoning. Due to my own feelings of guilt and powerlessness, I found it necessary to take intermittent breaks in my attempts to be with Anzor's rage and to help him express his anger rather than reenact it, manage his disappointments, and be able to seek support for his daughter's medical care. Despite his resurgence of resentment, I encouraged him to continue with the rehabilitation in order to gain a more realistic understanding of Malika's medical prognosis.

While in New York, we provided the opportunity for Anzor to speak with the families of other disabled children and, in that milieu, he seemed fortified to better confront the profound issues that fueled his anger. He expressed to me that in order for his family to survive during the war, he felt he had to shed his and his family's humanity for a while. He felt remorse for having submitted himself and his family to barbaric treatment by hiding in an underground tunnel to survive the Russian bombing in 2001. While watching the difficult and medically unattended birth of his daughter, he may have felt impotent for his inability to have access to medical resources to intervene and help his daughter. I empathized with his sense of helplessness of having to turn himself and his family into "underground animals" in order to survive the bombings, which must have felt devastatingly dehumanizing. Some of his understandable difficulty with more fully accepting his daughter's condition was somewhat assuaged by his being in a caring environment while in New York and having the support of other American parents of disabled children with similar experiences.

Anzor's sense of humiliation was not unique to other peoples subjected to genocide, where the aggression is driven to destroy their personhood, nor could his sense of shame in his survivor's psyche be wished away by our respectful ideas. The violence perpetrated in ethnic war and genocide is "purely to the identity and existence of the targeted group" (Hoffman, 2004).

It seemed that Anzor became somewhat more accepting of his daughter's condition. It may have been the cumulative influence of many physicians providing consistent medical information regarding his daughter's illness that contributed more to his ambivalent acceptance. Also, in our relationship, I functioned as a recognizing witness to his trauma. I would like to believe that "the being with" of our relationship was, in part, the agent of his change as well as my management of the strong countertransference responses our relationship evoked in me. From our initial meeting more than two years earlier, Anzor was able to take the leap of faith toward a relationship with me and I toward him. I finally was able to struggle through my feelings of guilt and powerlessness to surrender to empathic attunement while still holding on to my sense of self.

Countertransferentially, I went through what Anzor experienced in a more condensed period of time. When Anzor pulled out the tattered business card that I had given him in Grozny more than two years earlier from his shirt pocket and told me he had kept it close to his heart ever since, I felt an overwhelming sense of guilt, impotence, and responsibility for offering help and thereby exposing Anzor and his daughter to possible treatments that may never be available to them. The humiliation I felt at my inability to fix Malika's brain led me to reflect upon an earlier, concrete period of my own development where I felt inadequate.

During the middle of their stay, a medical internist expressed her anger that these Chechen children "should never have been brought to New York to receive medical treatment." This internist seemed to be expressing her anger and unprocessed feelings of guilt and remorse that we were able only to provide limited medical aid and could not erase the horrors that the Chechens had been exposed to nor their suffering from these subsequent medical illnesses as a result of the war.

By struggling through my own pain and working through my feelings of shame in therapy, I traveled to a more symbolic understanding and appreciation of what we did provide: helping to slowly release Anzor from his trauma by offering medical information on Malika's condition, sharing his pain, empathizing, and bearing witness to their trauma. As a result, I became better able to emotionally remain with Anzor through his anger, the redirection of his potentially self-destructive behavior, and his beginning to mourn the loss of the hope that his daughter would fully recover, and I helped diminish his magical beliefs in a cure for acceptance of the efficacy of realistic help. The intensity of Anzor's trauma experience, coupled with my initial failure of symbolic understanding of what our team did offer, made it initially difficult for me to navigate his turmoil and sustain myself through his maelstroms. This was a traumatic reenactment that eventually became a scene of post-traumatic growth for us both. Multimodal psychoanalytic understanding was a rich resource for accompanying this man in attempting to reshape his trauma experience as an object of memory as opposed to reenactment.

One antidote to compensate for the feeling of hopelessness that inevitably results from war may be the empowering feeling of "I can." Illusory as it was, Anzor's grandiose defense that "he can" nevertheless served him to survive the atrocities of the war, pursue a faith in improving his daughter's illness, and the tenacity to come to America. Both of us had to struggle through our grandiose sense of self in an attempt to overcome our mutual feelings of ineffectiveness to foster an acceptance of the limitations of my medical powers to cure, what we could medically provide, and the chronic nature of Malika's condition. Also, I unconsciously may have attempted to repair my long-held sense of impotence by a feeling of "I can" by going into the Second Chechen War to offer medical care. In both of us, our courage was a defense against feelings of helplessness. In order to submerge my anxious feelings of infectiousness, my grandiose defense, similar to Anzor's defense, helped me survive my childhood, and buoyed me into genuine accomplishments by becoming a physician and elite endurance athlete.

And like Anzor, my defense also ultimately got in my way as I had to discover more realistic acceptance. My counterphobic delusion of being warrior king which covered my sad feeling of helplessness had to be dragged into the golden middle so that I could accept my own limitations but still deliver the best medical care to Malika, in spite of the unavoidable limitations.

As Gerson (1996) has indicated, it is important for the analyst to work through shame in the transference, and that transference can be so shame-producing that it is avoided. Just as my mother did not recognize feelings of mine that were unimportant to her, I failed empathically in recognizing the feelings of Anzor. I overidentified with him and with the Chechens who were abandoned by the world. My feelings of being infectious all came sailing back for another slap in the face. My colluding with Anzor's feeling of shame that we could not fix Malika's brain prevented me from staying in the moment with Anzor's anger and attempting to work it through. The Chechen fight for freedom and independence resonated in me through my lifelong struggle not to be "colonized" by my mother's intrusiveness and to define my own "country" and sense of self. Indeed, similar to the Chechens who are portrayed historically as "terrorist" and "bandits" in their attempt to separate and be independent from Russia, I was seen as "bad" when attempting to separate and individuate from my mother, as she felt abandoned.

Our team needed to be constantly mindful of being emotionally present while maintaining enough distance to work with the visiting Chechen patients and families and not inflate goals. We needed to be aware of their expectations and of our own desire to meet those expectations. Through his boundless spirit and energy, Anzor was able to begin to reshape his trauma experience as an object of memory as opposed to reenactment, better reflect on and be less ambivalent on accepting Malika's medical condition, and become more realistic regarding her treatment and the limits of her recovery.

Conclusion: Balancing Hope with Limitations

As opposed to continuing the intergenerational legacy of trauma and entrapment, multimodal psychoanalytic and culturally sensitive medical and psychological care allowed our team to engender a sense of hope, wholeness, and the potential for post-traumatic growth in these children. While the odds are stacked against these survivors, we hoped that the progress initiated in New York would generate further growth when they returned to their homeland. It was a profound experience to balance the vicissitudes of the Chechens' hope against our limited promise of help, while exposing them to basic rights and freedoms they may never have. In working with these survivors, there was a vast opportunity for all involved to learn and grow.

Note

1 The Consolidated Appeals Process includes numerous United Nations organizations like the International Organization for Migration, the Red Cross, and the United Nations International Children Fund (UNICEF).

References

Auerhahn, N., & Laub, D. (1994). Annihilation and restoration: Post-traumatic memory as pathway and obstacle to recovery. *International Review of Psycho-Analysis*, *11*(3), 327–344.

Boulanger, G. (2005). From voyeur to witness: Recapturing symbolic function after massive psychic trauma. *Psychoanalytic Psychology*, *22*(1), 21–31.

Bromberg, P. M. (2000). Potholes on the royal road: Or is it an abyss? *Contemporary Psychoanalysis*, *36*(1), 5–28. https://doi.org/10.1080/00107530.2000.10747043

Cerfolio, N. (2009). Multimodal psychoanalytically informed aid work with children traumatized by the Chechen War. *The Journal of the American Academy of Psychoanalysis and Dynamic Psychiatry*, *37*(4), 587–603. https://doi.org/10.1521/jaap.2009.37.4.587

Cerfolio, N. (2016). Loss, surrender and spiritual awakening. *Palliative & Supportive Care*, *14*(6), 725–726. https://doi.org/10.1017/S1478951516000304

Cerfolio, N. (2020a, March). From Russia with anthrax. *Harmony*: Humanity Magazine, Program in Medical Humanities, The University of Arizona College of Medicine, Tucson, AZ.

Cerfolio, N. (2020b). The origins of terrorism: The obliteration of a sense of belonging. In R. C. Curtis (Ed.), *Belonging through a psychoanalytic lens*. Routledge.

Cerfolio, N. (2020c). Terrorism and the psychoanalytic origins. *The Journal of Psychohistory*, *47*(4), 256–274.

Cerfolio, N. (2023). *Psychoanalytic and spiritual perspectives on terrorism: Desire for destruction*. Routledge.

Cerfolio, N. (2024, April 18). How to alchemize a desire for destruction into connection: Spirituality and interconnectedness can be an antidote to terrorism and trauma. *Psychology Today*.

Davoine, F., & Gaudillière, J.-M. (2004). *History beyond trauma: Whereof one cannot speak, thereof one cannot stay silent*. Other Books.

Gerson, B. (1996). *The therapist as a person*. Analytic Press.

Goldfarb, A., & Litvinenko, M. (2007). *Death of a dissident: The poisoning of Alexander Litvinenko and the return of the KGB*. Free Press.

Grand, S. (1995). Incest and the intersubjective politics of knowing history. In J. L. Albert (Ed.), *Sexual Abuse Recalled*. Jason Aronson Inc.

Heim, C., & Nemeroff, C. B. (2001). The role of childhood trauma in the neurobiology of mood and anxiety disorders: Pre-clinical and clinical studies. *Biological Psychiatry*, *49*(12), 1023–1039.

Hoffman, E. (2004). *After such knowledge: Memory, history, and the legacy of the Holocaust*. PublicAffairs.

Klein, M. (1975). *Envy and gratitude and other works, 1946–1963*. Hogarth Press.

Konkov, F. (2001). Russia: An emptiness within. In J. D. Lindy & R. J. Lifton (Eds.), *Beyond invisible walls: The psychological legacy of Soviet trauma, Eastern European therapists and their patients* (pp. 120–139). Brunner-Routledge.

Krystal, H. (2004). Resilience: Accommodation and recovery. In D. Knafo (Ed.), *Living with terror, working with trauma: A clinician's handbook* (pp. 67–83). Jason Aronson.

Laub, D., & Auerhahn, N. (1989). Failed empathy: A central theme in the survivor's Holocaust experience. *Psychoanalytic Psychology*, *6*(4),377–400. https://doi.org/10.1037/0736-9735.6.4.377

Laub, D., & Auerhahn, N. (1993). Knowing and not knowing massive psychological trauma: Forms of traumatic memory. *International Journal of Psychoanalysis*, *74*(2), 287–302.

Lifton, R. J. (2022). Is Putin beyond influence? *Psychology Today*. https://www.psychologytoday.com/us/blog/the-guest-room/202203/is-putin-beyond-influence

Merridale, C. (2001). *Night of stone: Death and memory in twentieth-century Russia*. Penguin Books.

Nemeroff, C. B. (2004). Neurobiological consequences of childhood trauma. *Journal of Clinical Psychiatry*, *65* (suppl. 1), 18–27.

Person, E. S., & Klar, H. (1994). Establishing trauma: The difficulty distinguishing between memories and fantasies. *Journal of the American Psychological Association*, *42*(4), 1055–1081.

Politkovskaya, A. (2003). *A small corner of hell: Dispatches from Chechnya*. The University of Chicago Press.

Prince, R. (1998). Historical trauma: Psychohistorical reflections on the Holocaust. In J. Kestenberg and C. Kahn (Eds.), *Children surviving persecution: An International study of trauma and healing* (pp. 43–53). Praeger Books.

Rothe, E. (2008). A psychotherapy model for treating refugee children caught in the midst of catastrophic situations. *The Journal of the American Academy of Psychoanalysis and Dynamic Psychiatry*, *36*(4), 625–643. https://doi.org/10.1521/jaap.2008.36.4.625

Santostefano, S. (2004). *Child therapy in the great outdoors: A relational view*. The Analytic Press.

Seierstad, A. (2008). *The angel of Grozny*. Basic Books.

Ullman, C. (2006). Bearing witness: Across the barriers in society and in the clinic. *Psychoanalytic Dialogues*, *16*(2), 181–198.

Valent, P. (1998). Child survivors: A review. In J. Kestenberg & C. Kahn (Eds.), *An international study of trauma and healing* (pp. 109–123). Praeger Publishers.

Vinar, M. (2003). Subjectivity under extreme conditions. In J. A. Cancelmo, I. Tylim, J. Hoffenberg, & H. Myers (Eds.), *Terrorism and the psychoanalytic space* (pp. 171–172). Pace University Press.

Chapter 3

Social Psychoanalysis, Silencing, and Racial Violence

Roger Frie

Silencing of Racial Violence

In 2018, former Canadian Prime Minister Paul Martin was asked by a Black journalist what he knew about slavery in Canada. His response was as telling as it was instructive. Martin said that he grew up learning about the underground railroad, which helped escaped slaves from the United States find freedom in Canada between the 1830s and the 1860s. When asked whether he also knew that slavery existed as an institution, Martin responded, "I must plead guilty. I didn't realize that there was slavery in Canada anywhere" (Brown, 2018). In fact, the system of chattel slavery existed in what is now Canada for a period of over 200 years. The first recorded slave trade took place in 1628, and the legal and active practice of slavery continued until 1833, during which time thousands of enslaved Indigenous and African people provided labor for the new colonial economies.

Slavery was as brutal in Canada as it was south of the border in the United States. Yet the vast majority of Canadians continue to associate slavery with the plantations in the American South and remain ignorant of its existence in their own backyards. Given that the enslavement of Africans was common practice throughout centuries of British and French colonial rule in North America and the Caribbean, the question that must be asked is why Canadians would assume their country was exempt? It would require a kind of twisted logic, a paradoxical act of consciousness if you will, to acknowledge the reality of slavery throughout the British and French colonies yet deny its existence in Canada. Yet this is precisely what Canadian historians managed to do, despite the abundance of factual records.

DOI: 10.4324/9781003658382-4

While teaching at my university in Canada, each year I would begin by asking students how many were aware of their country's long history of slavery. When I first began asking this question, very few if any raised their hands. Over the course of nearly 20 years, the number of informed students increased, though only slightly. This may be in part a generational issue as elementary school children are now being taught this history in many, though by no means all, public schools. At the same time, many Black Canadians today continue to endure racial profiling by police, and Black citizens report being frequent targets of racism across the country (Maynard, 2017). As the celebrated Jamaican-born Canadian historian and poet Afua Cooper has pointedly stated, "If a Black history narrative makes Whites feel good, it is allowed to surface; if not, it is suppressed or buried" (2006, p. 8).

In 2021, another former Canadian prime minister, Jean Chrétien, gave a widely heard interview about his life and work in which he claimed that when he was minister of the Department of Indian Affairs from 1968 to 1974, he did not know about the abuse that existed in the nation's many Indian residential schools. "This problem was never mentioned when I was minister. Never" (Radio-Canada, 2021). A few years earlier in 2015, the Final Report of the Truth and Reconciliation Commission of Canada had revealed the full extent of the criminal history of Canada's Indian residential schools. For well over a century, the Canadian government practiced a policy of subjugation and forced assimilation against Indigenous peoples. It set up and funded Indian residential schools, which were run by Catholic and Protestant churches. Indigenous children as young as five years old were taken from their families and sent to faraway residential institutions where they were forbidden from speaking their language, endured rampant physical and sexual abuse, and suffered disease, malnutrition, and the consequences of gross neglect. Thousands died and were hastily buried, often without their families ever being notified. Despite these indisputable facts, when questioned in his interview, Chrétien went on to draw a direct comparison between his own experience of attending a conventional Quebec college boarding school and that of Indigenous children who were forced to attend residential schools. "I ate baked beans and oatmeal. And to be sure, it was hard living in a boarding school, extremely hard" (Radio-Canada, 2021). Chrétien added that while he didn't enjoy sleeping in a dorm with 200 others, neither did he ever experience any problems, thereby effectively putting his own experiences and those of residential school survivors on the same plane.

Indigenous leaders in Canada were saddened and outraged by Chrétien's comments and with good reason. It took until 1997 before the last residential school in Canada was closed. The traumatic effects of this violently racist history are still evident for the 60,000 residential school survivors living in Canada today. Many First Nations continue to lack access to drinkable water, adequate housing, healthcare, and education. Substance abuse and suicide are widespread, especially among younger Indigenous generations. In the year 2017, Canada's Indigenous citizens accounted for a little over 4% of the nation's overall population, yet made up 26% of its prison population. Even more alarming is the fact that Indigenous youth today make up only 8% of Canada's youth population, yet account for 46% of all admissions to youth correctional services. This is despite the fact that crime rates fell in the previous decades (Office of the Correctional Investigator, 2017).

In 2015 the Truth and Reconciliation Committee concluded that Canada's system of Indian residential schools and its colonial relationship to Indigenous peoples amounted to cultural genocide. In 2019, the National Inquiry into Murdered and Missing Indigenous Women and Girls went a step further to conclude that genocide had been committed. It's hard to argue with these conclusions, though many have and for different reasons. In 1883, Canada's first prime minister, John A. Macdonald, stood up in the House of Commons and notoriously argued for the removal of Indigenous children from their so-called savage parents so they could learn the ways of so-called civilized White men. In 1920, despite ample evidence of the staggering loss of Indigenous life at residential schools, Deputy Minister of Indian Affairs Duncan Campbell Scott insisted that the high mortality rate "does not justify a change in the policy of this Department, which is geared towards a final solution of our Indian Problem" (BC Teachers' Federation, 2015).[1] The cruel and undeniable reality is that Indigenous peoples were subjugated, pushed off their land, deprived of food, killed in large numbers, and forced to send their children to institutions that implemented genocidal policies.

It may be tempting to view these two examples of Canada's deeply racist past as an aberration. Afterall, this history doesn't conform with the popular image of Canada as a nation that is guided by tolerance and respect for diversity. We are not only forced to question our perceived understanding of Canada; we also need to ask how it has been possible for an ostensibly progressive nation to engage in such willful denial of its own history. It is important to emphasize that Paul Martin and Jean Chrétien were liberal prime ministers, not right-wing firebrands. They served consecutive terms and together governed Canada from 1993 to 2006. Martin and Chrétien are members of an older generation, but their views are by no means unusual. Indeed, while their responses are jarring, their stance represents the collective silencing of Canada's White majority toward the historical realities of racial violence experienced by Black and Indigenous people in Canada (Frie, 2026).

To be sure, from my vantage point as a White, male Canadian professor and psychoanalyst living in the multicultural and majority Asian city of Vancouver, it can sometimes feel as though I reside in a place apart from the right-wing populism and extremism that is shaping the political discourse in countries around the globe. And indeed, Canada is often perceived as a nation that is uniquely defined by its multiculturalism. There is some truth to this, and for the moment at least, Canada's political culture has enabled it to negotiate some of the ideological battles currently being waged in other countries. But there are undeniable cracks in this narrative, which obligate us to look for counter narratives.

From the perspective of its U.S. neighbor, Canada is often granted the status of a "kinder, gentler place," one that is supposedly free of the racist attitudes seen south of the border. It's a nice narrative, one that White Canadians like myself are only too eager to embrace. It makes us feel good, and who doesn't like to feel good? In fact, there are many White Canadians today that still associate racism with what happens "south of the border." In general, we attend to narratives and versions of history that match how we'd like to be seen and how we'd like to think about ourselves. For many White Canadians, racism in Canada is an inconvenient truth or dissonant reality. But as the examples I have shared suggest, once we are able to challenge the narratives we are told and only too ready to accept, then the legacy of Canada's racial violence and its European colonial past becomes evident for all to see.

The revelation disrupts the denial and dissociation that often obscures racial harm, necessitating a crucial reassessment of responsibility and the frameworks through which so-called White identity in Canada is constructed and understood.

From a psychoanalytic perspective, the question that must be asked is not only how to understand the process of collective silencing I have described but also how to break out of the cycle of self-enclosed narratives that serve the needs of a White majority to the detriment of Black and Indigenous minorities who continue to be disadvantaged and discriminated against. These were precisely the kinds of questions that Erich Fromm, the mid-century Jewish-German sociologist and psychoanalyst, sought to explore. Fromm was concerned above all with how a society could maintain an oppressive status quo, despite the obvious and evident harm such a system created.

Fromm stands out in the history of psychoanalysis. He was one of very few analysts to speak openly about the dangers of fascism while it was still emerging in the late 1930s (Fromm, 1941), and he later addressed the impact of racism in the United States at a time when most mainstream analysts believed that the intrapsychic realm should be the sole focus of their work (Fromm, 1964). The fundamental difference in outlook between Fromm's progressive and emancipatory approach and the more conservative mainstream effectively pushed him to the peripheries of the profession. It led to the widespread neglect, if not denial, of his ideas by fellow psychoanalysts. In the discussion that follows, I will turn to Fromm's work to examine how his legacy can help us to understand the process of silencing and what it can tell us about establishing potential avenues for change—change that is both individual and social in nature. It will be helpful to begin with some background on who Fromm was and how he came to develop an approach that became known as social psychoanalysis. Throughout my discussion I will refer back to the examples of silencing.

Social Psychoanalysis

Throughout his long career, Fromm argued that it was essential for psychoanalysis to integrate an understanding of the individual patient with the recognition of the role played by social forces in the shaping of all experience (Frie, 2024). In developing this approach, Fromm drew on his academic training in sociology and clinical training in psychoanalysis. Fromm received his doctorate in sociology with Alfred Weber (the brother of Max Weber) at the University of Heidelberg in 1922, and he graduated from the Berlin Psychoanalytic Institute, where he was analyzed by Hanns Sachs and became a full member of the German Psychoanalytic Association or DPG in 1930.

In 1929, Fromm gave a lecture in Frankfurt on "Psychoanalysis and Sociology," which was a preliminary attempt to create a synthesis between Freud and Marx. This essay demonstrates a key theme in his early work—namely, understanding and explaining the process of socialization. Fromm's innovative work brought him to the attention of Max Horkheimer, the director of Frankfurt's Institute for Social Research, who recognized Fromm's psychoanalytic prowess. Horkheimer made Fromm the director of social psychology and psychoanalysis, a tenured position that he held for ten years. Under the auspices of the Institute, Fromm began his project of integrating Marxism and psychoanalysis.

The rise of Hitler and the Nazi Party and their election to power in Germany in 1933 led Fromm, who was both Jewish and a Marxist, to escape first to Switzerland and then to the United States (Frie, 2024). He arrived in New York in 1934. Throughout the writings he undertook in the 1930s in Germany, Switzerland, and the United States, Fromm sought to show how people are shaped by social and cultural forces. Fromm's approach was evident in a number of different works from the period, including *The Dogma of Christ* (1930) in which he traced the development of religious belief. In brief, Fromm argued that changes in individual belief are as a result of broader changes that take place at the level of society, thus inverting the traditional focus on the individual. His aim was to shed light on the determinative role of social factors. In a similar sense, Fromm maintained that the analysis of group phenomena should not be explained through analogy to the neurotic symptom formation in individuals. Rather, it should focus on the role of the societal forces.

In the process of laying out his social psychoanalytic approach, Fromm became increasingly critical of Freudian psychoanalysis and the intrapsychic model of mind. As Fromm wrote to his colleague Karl August Wittfogel in 1936,

> Those urges which motivate social activities are not, as Freud supposes, sublimations of sexual instincts, but rather products of social processes. These urges … are not to be understood biologically, but rather as in the context of the practice of social living. … Freud has wrongly based psychology totally on natural factors.
>
> (Cited in Funk, 2019, p. 53)

This line of thinking found full expression in Fromm's article "Man's Impulse Structure and Its Relation to Culture" from 1937. Fromm focused above all on the limitations that followed from Freud's drive theory. He took issue with Freud's biologically determined account of human nature which, he argued, was unable to account for social and cultural factors in the shaping of the person, and he altogether rejected Freud's psychology of women, which he saw as effectively a means of rationalizing patriarchy.[2]

Fromm (2010c/1937) explained the intertwining of the individual person and society as follows:

> Society and the individual are not "opposite" to each other. *Society is nothing but living, concrete individuals, and the individual exists only as a social human being*. His individual life practice is necessarily determined by the life practice of his society or class and, in the last analysis, by the manner of production of his society, that is, how this society produces, how it is organized to satisfy the needs of its members. The differences in the manner of production and life of various societies or classes lead to the development of different character structures typical of the particular society. Various societies differ from each other not only in differences in manner of production and social and political organization but also in that their people exhibit a typical character structure despite all individual differences. We shall call this "*the socially typical character*."
>
> (p. 58, italics in original)

Fromm thus positioned the person within social, cultural, and political relations in order to reveal the effect of these forces on human well-being. Drawing on his understanding of Marx, Fromm suggested that it was by virtue of our participation in society that we learned to contain thoughts and feelings that might otherwise challenge the status quo. In this way, society inscribed pathology into human relationships. For Fromm, therefore, the goal of psychoanalysis was never simply to adapt to society's needs but to help us embrace a more grounded and ethically centered stance, in essence, to live soundly against the stream.

As Fromm (1949) would famously remark in a later work,

> It is the function of social character to shape the energies of the members of society in such a way that their behavior is not left to conscious decisions whether or not to follow the social pattern but that *people want to act as they have to act*.
>
> (p. 5, italics in original)

The point, for Fromm, was that society was always at work in the person. According to Fromm, society shaped individuals to match the needs of the social, cultural, economic, and political contexts in which they live and work. This process takes place through the production of socially necessary character types that harness the energies of individuals and enable society to function.

Social Unconscious and Social Filters

The challenge for psychoanalysis is to recognize the way in which pathologies of domination and power in social, cultural, economic and political interactions are inscribed into psychological life. Yet all too often, psychoanalysis neglects the role of social factors. As Fromm demonstrates, social systems cannot be separated from individual well-being; they are the ground out of which well-being emerges. This argument is as relevant today as when Fromm (1944) first proposed it:

> The psychoanalyst is not only concerned with the readjustment of the neurotic individual to his given society. His task must be also to recognize that the individual's ideal of normalcy may contradict the aim of the full realization of himself as a human being.
>
> (p. 384)

The point is that our ideal of normalcy is socially constructed and serves the needs of the society or the group in which we participate.

If we turn back to the two examples of silencing that I shared at the start of the chapter, we can see that both Martin and Chrétien expressed a stance of dissociation and denial respectively. The silence that their responses to the interviewers embodied were not only representative of their personal views. Rather, their personal views were themselves reflective of the collective needs of the White majority in Canada, which has long sought to silence Canada's history of racial violence and thus maintain the status quo.

Seen from this perspective, psychoanalysis is not just seeking the amelioration of individual suffering. It needs to attend to the social structures that give rise to suffering. Hence, Fromm argues for a reversal of sorts. It is not enough to be concerned simply with individual pathology. He suggests that psychoanalysts also need to address the "pathology of contemporary Western society" – namely, with the "pathology of normalcy" (Fromm, 1990/1955). The question remains, if the psychological processes that shape suffering are outside of the patient's awareness, residing in the unconscious, how might we attend to this problem? Here it is important to note that for Fromm, the unconscious is never strictly individual but rather is interwoven with society. Fromm (2000/1959) maintains,

> If we really want to understand the unconscious ... that part which exists and which the social filter, as I call it, does not permit to come into awareness, then indeed we have to transcend the frame of reference of our society. I would put it this way: We can understand the unconscious fully only if we are critical and aware of the limitations of our own culture and the patterns of our society. If we are caught in them like everybody else, then indeed we cannot really understand.... The critical understanding and awareness of the fiction in the social pattern in which we live is a very essential condition for the full awareness of the dissociated part of another person.
>
> (p. 180)

To begin to grasp unconscious psychological processes, therefore, it is not enough to focus only on the individual patient's dynamic dissociations. Individual psychological processes *always* need to be understood in connection to broader social structures and forces. What this implies, in short, is that we work to understand and acknowledge our embeddedness and to discover how and why we recreate the world in which we find ourselves. Differently expressed, psychoanalytic understanding is not simply the product of the individual mind, or even of two interacting minds but, rather, is grounded in an understanding of how we exist in social and cultural patterns of interaction and meaning. This is what the cultural psychologist Philip Cushman (1995) suggests when he states,

> The unconscious is not an interior thing, but part of the patient's social landscape that contains potential feelings, thoughts, and experiences that are not able to show up because they lie on the other side of the patient's horizon of understanding.
>
> (p. 307)

The reason certain ideas and feelings remain hidden and out of reach points to the role of social filters. Their purpose is to prevent the emergence into conscious awareness of ideas or feelings that might threaten the social status quo and upend the social structures on which the status quo depends. Fromm suggests that ideology functions to shape individuals in such a manner that they adhere to social norms and practices even to the detriment of their own well-being. The process of being shaped by ideology is implicit or unconscious and can take place variously through the family, community, education, and the media. In short, social filters help to quell critical thinking about the way in which society functions. The emancipatory potential of Fromm's theory lies in its attempt to bring to light, reveal, and disclose those ideas and feelings that have been denied, dissociated, and silenced and thus create possibilities for liberatory social change.

In laying out his approach, Fromm (1962) takes pains to distinguish himself from Freud:

> Freud was mainly concerned with the uncovering of the individual unconscious. While he assumed that society enforced repressions, these were repressions of instinctual forces—and not the social repressions that really matter—the repressions of awareness of social contradictions, socially produced suffering .... Freudian psychoanalysis has shown that it is possible to some degree to make the individual unconscious conscious without touching the social

> unconscious. However, it follows … that any de-repression that excludes the social sphere must remain limited. The full awareness of what has been repressed is possible only if it transcends the individual realm, and if the process includes the analysis of the social unconscious.
>
> (Fromm, 1962, pp. 123–124)

The point for Fromm is that without an awareness of the role played by the social unconscious and social filters in maintaining the status quo, "socially conditioned taboos and restrictions must appear 'natural'" (Fromm, 1962, p. 124). This process thus necessarily involves the "understanding of social dynamics and the critical appraisal of one's own society." Fromm's notions of the social unconscious and social filters are helpful for understanding the silencing, dissociation, and denial in regard to the history of slavery and Indigenous genocide in Canada. We can see the ways in which social filters among majority White Canadians sought to silence any critical and conscious awareness of this history of deep racial injustice.[3] This process was undoubtedly variously motivated, but several possible reasons stand out: for some members of the White majority in Canada, speaking out about this silenced history is not seen as relevant because the history of violence is believed to have conformed with the colonial and racist perspectives that were held by the majority of White Canadians at the time they occurred; for others, this history does not conform with how many members of the White majority have come to see themselves, especially in relation to their nation's multiculturalism, and in contrast to the White majority in the United States, who are identified with their nation's more obvious racist history.

In both cases, social filters help to sustain the status quo of White supremacy, even as contemporary Canadian society celebrates its diversity and tolerance. What needs to be emphasized is that the viewpoints articulated by Paul Martin and Jean Chrétien should be understood as representing wider social patterns in Canadian society that are historically entrenched and not easily dislodged. The point is that from the social psychoanalytic perspective articulated by Fromm, change cannot come about only at the individual level, as important as that is. Rather, change begins through critical engagement with Canada's long history of structural racism and through the recognition that racial discrimination continues to shape the lives of Black and Indigenous peoples today.

Being able to take such a critical viewpoint requires a willingness to challenge accepted patterns of thinking and acting in order to disclose that which has remained silenced, in effect to listen to the voices of victims and survivors and to articulate stories that have yet to be told. This implies creating and restoring a space for emergent views and voices rather than normalizing or reinscribing the status quo.

Learning to challenge the status quo and reflecting critically on how society functions is essential. Without this social understanding, the psychoanalytic process easily devolves into a form of social adjustment. As Fromm (1990/1955) reminds us,

> Mental health cannot be defined in terms of the "adjustment" of the individual to his society, but, on the contrary, that it must be defined in terms of the adjustment of society to the needs of man, of its role in furthering or hindering the development of mental health. Whether or not the individual is healthy, is primarily not an individual matter, but depends on the structure of his society. A healthy society furthers man's capacity to love his fellow men, to work creatively, to develop his reason and objectivity, to have a sense of self which is based on the experience of his own productive powers. An unhealthy society is one which creates mutual hostility, distrust, which transforms man into an instrument of use and exploitation for others, which deprives him of a sense of self, except inasmuch as he submits to others or becomes an automaton.
>
> (p. 70)

Critique of Social Adaptation

In a move that may initially seem surprising to the reader, Fromm located an example of social adjustment in the work of his close colleague Harry Stack Sullivan. When Fromm was developing his critical perspective on Sullivan's work, he had already moved to Mexico City, where he lived and worked from 1950 through the early 1970s. This distance enabled him to develop a critical perspective on the social structures underpinning postwar-American society and psychoanalysis.

While praising the importance of Sullivan's work, Fromm also criticized him for developing theories of the self that were a reflection of the way in which modern capitalist society shaped human experience (Frie, 2014; Frie and Sauvayre, 2022). As Fromm (1990/1955) wrote,

> Our current psychiatric definitions of mental health stress those qualities which are part of the alienated social character of our time: adjustment, co-operativeness, aggressiveness, tolerance, ambition.... Even one of the most profound and brilliant psychoanalysts of our period, H. S. Sullivan, was influenced in his theoretical concepts by the all-pervasive alienation. Just because of his eminence and the important contribution he made to psychiatry, it will be enlightening to dwell somewhat on this point. Sullivan took the fact that the alienated person lacks a feeling of selfhood and experiences himself in terms of a response to the expectation of others, as part of human nature, just as Freud had taken the competitiveness characteristic of the beginning of the century as a natural phenomenon.
>
> (p. 193)

In particular, Fromm argued that two of Sullivan's key concepts, the "delusion of unique individuality" and the "need for personal security," were for all intents and purposes, a concretization of cultural patterns at the time. Thus, according to Fromm, rather than recognize the dangers of adjustment to society or the effects of alienation caused by social forces, Sullivan assumed that the lack of a feeling of selfhood and the need for personal security against anxiety was a part of human nature. For Fromm (1990/1955), by contrast, "life, in its mental and spiritual aspects, is by necessity insecure and uncertainty" (p. 196).

My aim here is not to enter into a discussion of Sullivan's ideas, many of which are highly applicable to therapeutic work.[4] Rather, what I want to consider is how Sullivan's account of the place of society in relation to human experience highlights the problematic issue of social adaptation (or adjustment—the term used by Fromm). According to Sullivan (1940), the successful negotiation of personality development includes "the freedom of personal initiative that represents a comfortable adaptation of one's personal situation to the circumstances that characterize the social order of which one is a part" (p. 57). Despite Sullivan's progressive impulse, which was evidenced in his analysis and critique of racism (Sullivan, 1964) and antisemitism (Sullivan, 1938) in the United States, the obvious ambiguity with which he treated the issue of social adaptation is hard to question. Indeed, interpersonal psychoanalysts have themselves (cf. Greenberg & Mitchell, 1983, p. 112) long sought to make sense of this statement. Why would Sullivan maintain a belief that adaptation to society's social order was a marker of successful personality development?

As a gay man living in a strongly homophobic society, Sullivan certainly knew what it meant to be "othered," and he was strongly critical of social institutions that made prejudice possible. However, with the benefit of hindsight, we also might wonder whether it was precisely Sullivan's understanding of the effects of prejudice that led him to observe the psychological ease of individuals who conformed to society's expectations. The interpersonal analyst Edgar Levenson (1992) adds another perspective when he writes,

> Sullivan felt clearly there was an external reality, separate from the patient and therapist and the possibility of consensual validation. It was the function of the therapist to help the patient give up his/her distortions and enter the real world. This world was, itself, a matter of consensual validation; inasmuch as Sullivan seemed to believe that there was a community of people living without major distortions in their world. For Sullivan getting well, being normal, was seeing the world the way it was—which was the way normal people saw it. It was this conservatism, this acceptance of the status quo which offended Erich Fromm and caused him to accuse Sullivan of selling out to Mammon. Sullivan apparently felt that being normal—being able to have intimate relationships, avoiding terrible loneliness—was a greater imperative than eschewing seduction by a marketing culture. About that, Sullivan apparently couldn't have cared less.
>
> (p. 459)

In contrast to Sullivan, Fromm conveyed no ambiguity with respect to the negative effects of social adaptation. Indeed, he equated adaptation with conformism—in short, with a kind of neurotic relatedness that could and must be resisted. For Fromm, the achievement of well-being was dependent upon revealing and resisting social and cultural forces that fostered and maintained inequality. Whereas Sullivan viewed human development in a social interactional context, Fromm's critique of social mores and institutions derived from his Marxist background and pointed to the fact that well-being was not a value-neutral undertaking but, rather, an inherently political affair.

Integrating a Critical Perspective

I have suggested, drawing on Fromm, that the psychoanalyst must develop a critical awareness of how social and political forces shape psychological life. Having examined Fromm's work, I want to come full circle and ask what it means to locate oneself in systems of oppression, to hear voices that have been silenced, and discover the limits of what one knows. What might it mean for me, as a majority White psychoanalyst in Canada, to practice in a society with a long and deep history of racial violence? For example, how might I work with or be of help to my Indigenous patients? At a minimum, the direct link between my patients' suffering and the societal racial violence that Indigenous people endured must be recognized; it cannot be reduced to libidinal drives or be understood as an individual "failure" to adapt to the effects of intergenerational trauma. But my responsibility goes much further.

As a majority White, male Canadian I am a participant and beneficiary of the structural racism that is the cause of my patients' suffering. I am offered societal privileges that are not shared by my patients, privileges that I may take for granted and not be aware of by virtue of my identity. Unless I can recognize my own subject position, no matter how uncomfortable it may make me feel, I simply continue to exacerbate the existing discriminatory dynamics. There is no easy resolution. Even when I acknowledge my social position and the benefits that I accrue by virtue of being White, the inequities that are created and sustained by structural racism remain. Indeed, they reappear, week after week, shaping my patients' experiences and determining what I am able to see and hear at any given moment. This recognition requires me to be aware of the realities of living in a systemically racist society on an ongoing basis. There is no point of resolution at which I am suddenly absolved on my responsibility to engage critically with my place in society or the inherently unequal ways in which that society functions, just as there is also no resolution for Indigenous residential school survivors and their descendants from the traumas created by the history of racial violence committed against them.

Fromm was asking us, in effect, to think critically about how our societies function, a process that necessitated the recognition of the social unconscious and the challenges involved in creating change. I have suggested that the process of change emerges out of a critical engagement with how we develop in and are shaped by social structures. This viewpoint has important implications. It requires us to see psychological life through the lens of society, culture, and politics and to contest the status quo. Achieving a state of well-being may require nothing less than the transformation of our social system into one in which just and compassionate relations with others can be realized. This can be achieved both through the lens applied in our individual clinical work and through how we teach and train future psychoanalysts to engage with the impact and reality of the social unconscious.

When I read Fromm's work today, I often look for contemporary parallels. The work of Cushman provides one such example, and I want to conclude by quoting Cushman since I believe that what he argued was directly relevant to Fromm's project (see also Layton, 2024). According to Cushman (2019),

> The reason to work as a psychotherapist is not … simply to help make conscious and/or attenuate the individual suffering of one's patients. The reason to work as a therapist is also to help patients become aware of the socio-political causes of their suffering, better understand the connections between the shape of their social world and the human suffering that it causes, and develop the political ideas and moral energy necessary to change that world. For me, that means assisting patients in becoming more politically progressive.… If our work isn't to prepare our patients to bring on and work toward a better world, what good is it? If therapists don't think in a more political—and more politically progressive—manner, and help others prepare themselves for becoming more active and effective in causes of the left, it is likely very few others will.
>
> (pp. 119–120)

As if to answer his critics, those who might look askance at the notion that politics is always and already in the consulting room, Cushman (2019) adds,

> I do not mean we should argue with our patients about elections and political parties, and I do not mean we should brand some actions—or worse yet, some people—as immoral. But we should

> keep in mind that the power relations of our society are always already influencing us, and the moral understandings that give shape to those relations are embodied by us and are being expressed by us, one way or another.
>
> (p. 120)

The point is that a culture of psychoanalysis that emphasizes the inner self neglects our existence in a community of shared values. Fromm believed that when the psychoanalyst focuses chiefly on the intrapsychic realm of the patient, or on the conscious and unconscious dynamics of the interaction between the analyst and patient, then the impact of social values, norms, and concepts are neglected. As a result, psychological experience tends to be viewed in isolation from the very contexts that define and limit it.

I have suggested that psychoanalysis is of value precisely when it is grounded in a socially conscious awareness and can work toward fostering well-being on both an individual and societal level. In a world that is increasingly riven by social and political crises, where the threat of authoritarian governments, vast economic disparities, and ecological disasters continues to expand, the efficacy of psychoanalysis is dependent upon establishing and maintaining an ethical framework that can bring about social transformation, not just social adaptation.

Notes

1 Scott's notorious statement was made in the context of a discussion about the effects of Indian residential schools on the health of Indigenous children. The full statement reads,

> It is readily acknowledged that Indian children lose their natural resistance to illness by habitating so closely in these schools, and that they die at a much higher rate than in their villages. But this alone does not justify a change in the policy of this Department, which is being geared towards the final solution of our Indian Problem.
>
> (BC Teachers' Federation, 2015)

2 Not surprisingly, perhaps, Fromm's critical viewpoint found little sympathy among his Freudian colleagues. When Fromm submitted "Man's Impulse Structure and Its Relation to Culture" for publication to the *Journal of the Institute for Social Research*, it was soundly rejected. Fromm's evolving

understanding of psychoanalysis clashed with the increasingly orthodox Freudian position represented by the Institute. Fromm and Horkheimer had long enjoyed a cordial relationship, and Fromm played a role in helping the Institute move from their temporary exile in Geneva to a more permanent home at Columbia University. But growing differences in their interpretations of Marx and Freud, made worse by Fromm's acrimonious interactions with Theodore Adorno, meant that there was little future for him at the Institute. As a result, after Fromm left in 1939, he was largely written out of the history of the Institute for Social Research, despite his formative early role as director of social psychology and psychoanalysis (Frie, 2024).

3 I have described a similar process of silencing within German families during the postwar decades regarding the participation of relatives in the Nazi past. This process was frequently motivated by attempts to keep knowledge of responsibility for the Holocaust at bay (Frie, 2017).

4 My concern here is less with Sullivan's ideas per se, which are both valuable and highly applicable in clinical contexts, than with the rationale for Fromm's critique. For an overview of Sullivan's work, see Cushman, 1995, pp. 169–185, and Greenberg and Mitchell, 1983, pp. 79–115.

Bibliography

BC Teachers' Federation (2015). *Project of heart: Illuminating the history of Indian Residential Schools in BC*. British Columbia Teacher's Foundation.

Brown, K. (2018, June 28). Canada's slavery secret: The whitewashing of 200 years of enslavement. *CBC Ideas Podcast*. https://www.cbc.ca/radio/ideas/canada-s-slavery-secret-the-whitewashing-of-200-years-of-enslavement-1.4726313

Cooper, A. (2006). *The hanging of Angélique: The untold story of Canadian slavery and the burning of Montreal*. HarperCollins.

Cushman, P. (1995). *Constructing the self, constructing America: A cultural history of psychotherapy*. Addison-Wesley.

Cushman, P. (2019). *Travels with the self: Interpreting psychology as cultural history*. Routledge.

Frie, R. (2014). What is cultural psychoanalysis? Psychoanalytic anthropology and the interpersonal tradition. *Contemporary Psychoanalysis*, *50*(3), 371–394. https://doi.org/10.1080/00107530.2014.895929

Frie, R. (2017). *Not in my family: German memory and responsibility after the Holocaust*. Oxford University Press.

Frie, R. (2024). *Edge of catastrophe: Erich Fromm, fascism, and the Holocaust*. Oxford University Press.

Frie, R. (2026). *Wounds of silence: Legacies of genocide and racial violence*. Oxford University Press.

Frie, R., and Sauvayre, P. (Eds.) (2022). *Culture, politics and race in the making of interpersonal psychoanalysis: Breaking boundaries*. Routledge.

Fromm, E. (1941). *Escape from freedom*. Farrar & Rinehart, Inc.

Fromm, E. (1944). Individual and social origins of neurosis. *American Sociological Review*, *9*(4), 380–384.

Fromm, E. (1949). Psychoanalytic characterology and its application to the understanding of culture. In S. S. Sargent & M. W. Smith (Eds.), *Culture and personality* (pp. 1–12). Viking Fund.

Fromm, E. (1962). *Beyond the chains of illusion: My encounter with Marx and Freud*. Abacus.

Fromm, E. (1963). The dogma of Christ. In E. Fromm (Ed.), *The dogma of Christ and other essays on religion, psychology, and culture* (pp. 15–94). Holt, Rinehart and Winston. (Original work published 1930)

Fromm, E. (1964). *The heart of man: Its genius for good and evil*. Harper & Row.

Fromm, E. (1989). Psychoanalysis and sociology. In S. E. Bronner & D. Kellner (Eds.), *Critical theory and society: A reader* (pp. 37–39). Routledge. (Original work published 1929)

Fromm, E. (1990). *The sane society*. Holt, Rinehart and Winston. (Original work published 1955)

Fromm, E. (2000). Dealing with the unconscious in psychotherapeutic practice. *International Forum of Psychoanalysis*, *9*(3–4), 167–186. (Original work publisehed 1959)

Fromm, E. (2010a). Man's impulse structure and its relation to culture. In R. Funk (Ed.), *Beyond Freud: From individual to social psychology* (pp. 17–74). American Mental Health Foundation. (Original work published 1937).

Fromm, E. (2010b). *The heart of man: Its genius for good and evil*. American Mental Health Foundation Books. (Original work published 1964).

Fromm, E. (2010c). The social determination of psychoanalytic theory. In R. Funk (Ed.), *The essential Fromm: Life between having and being* (p. 58). Bloomsbury Academic. (Original work published 1937).

Funk, R. (2019). *Life itself is an art: The life and work of Erich Fromm*. Bloomsbury Academic.

Greenberg, J., & Mitchell, S. A. (1983). *Object relations in psychoanalytic theory*. Harvard University Press.

Layton, L. (2024). Erich Fromm: Ancestor of social psychoanalytic practice. *Psychoanalytic Inquiry*, *44*(1), 26–36.

Levenson, E. A. (1992). From interpersonal psychiatry to interpersonal psychoanalysis. *Contemporary Psychoanalysis*, *28*(3), 450–466.

Maynard, R. (2017). *Policing Black lives: State violence in Canada from slavery to the present*. Fernwood Press.

Office of the Correctional Investigator. (2017). Annual report 2016–2017. https://oci-bec.gc.ca/en/content/annual-report-office-correctional-investigator-2016-2017

Radio-Canada. (2021, October 25). Jean Chrétien says he never heard about abuse in residential schools while he was minister. https://ici.radio-canada.ca/rci/en/news/1834305/jean-chretien-says-he-never-heard-about-abuse-in-residential-schools-while-he-was-minister

Sullivan, H. S. (1938). Antisemitism. *Psychiatry: Journal of the Biology and the Pathology of Interpersonal Relations*, *1*, 593–598.

Sullivan, H. S. (1940). *Conceptions of modern psychiatry*. Norton.

Sullivan, H. S. (1964). Discussion of the case of Warren Wall. In P. Mullahy (Ed.), *The fusion of psychiatry and social science* (pp. 100–107). Norton & Company. (Original work published 1940).

Chapter 4

Traveling Through Time

A Group Intervention in Northern Ireland[1]

M. Gerard Fromm

The Troubles

A number of years ago, several members of the International Dialogue Initiative (IDI) were invited to design and facilitate a set of meetings to address an outbreak of violence in Belfast, the capital of Northern Ireland. Over the course of 30 years, sectarian violence between Protestants and Catholics—a period known as The Troubles—had led to more than 3,500 deaths. This was not only a religious conflict; it was also a political one, dating at least as far back as the Irish War of Independence in the early part of the 20th century. One side, predominantly Catholic, wanted to unite (or they would say "reunite") Northern Ireland with the Republic of Ireland; the other side, predominantly Protestant, wanted Northern Ireland to remain part of the United Kingdom. There is a much longer history of oppression and conflict between the UK and Ireland, including the devastating famine of the mid-1800s, which many historians see as in part the result of callous mismanagement by British overlords.

Beginning in the early 1980s, a lengthy, risky, and turbulent dialogue process was begun, culminating in the Good Friday Agreement of 1998. This, more or less, ended the fighting and established a power-sharing government (Strozier, 2025). The Agreement has held for more than two decades, though outbreaks of violence do occur periodically. At the time of this intervention, the conflict had to do, at least overtly, with escalating tensions about the protocol for flying the Union flag. Given this terrible history, such a resurgence of violence is always of great concern.

DOI: 10.4324/9781003658382-5

The Retreat

The retreat designed by members of the IDI brought together high-level representatives from all five of Northern Ireland's major political parties as well as civic leaders from various segments of society—senior police officers, the Gaelic Athletic Association, clergy, a business executive, and leaders of NGOs, including a representative of a victims' organization. Organized by an ecumenical group, the meeting was held over two days at a remote retreat house, called Corrymeela, on the north coast. Five formal 1.5-hour sessions took place over this time; members, the ecumenical group, and the facilitating team shared meals and engaged informally outside the sessions. There were 21 invited participants and a team of 5 IDI facilitators, of which I was one.

The International Dialogue Initiative

The team was led by Dr. Vamik Volkan (2020), whose study of societal conflict was galvanized by two moments: the first when his medical school friend was killed in the civil war in Cyprus; the second when Anwar Sadat, the then president of Egypt, said that the trouble between Arabs and Israelis was "70% psychological." Dr. Volkan, while carrying on a psychoanalytic practice, immersed himself in projects related to the psychological understanding of societal conflict, working over long periods of time with Turks and Kurds, Israelis and Arabs, Estonians and Russians, among others. Later, as a scholar at the Erikson Institute of the Austen Riggs Center, he founded the IDI.

The IDI (Volkan et al., 2023) is now a small independent group of professionals from various nations and various disciplines whose task is to develop psychological understanding and interventions to address large-group conflict. It's actually a network of support, learning and consultation for the work that individual members carry out. The Northern Ireland intervention, however, was taken up by the IDI as a collective and carried out by an IDI team. Based on Dr. Volkan's work, the IDI develops concepts like large-group identity, the intergenerational transmission of trauma, and societal regression, as well as his Tree Model methodology, which works with the dynamics of dialogue between enemy groups and, ideally, helps to prepare the ground for future negotiations.

The Task

At Corrymeela, the agreed-upon task was to explore and diagnose underlying psychological obstacles to a more peaceful and stable Northern Ireland. The IDI team's aim was not to focus on individual dynamics, except to the degree that they might represent the larger group and societal dynamic. Participants in this kind of meeting—because they are embedded in the identity of their groups and because the immediate group dynamic pushes for it—inevitably function as informal spokespersons for the groups they represent. By listening to personal stories and observing interactions among the participants, the team tried to understand, name, and describe various processes that were very likely occurring in and between large groups in Northern Ireland: Catholics and Protestants, Unionists and Nationalists, and various political and community organizations.

Our effort—a profoundly psychoanalytic one—was to help participants go beyond political statements and talk openly about emotional issues that might be very difficult to speak about, issues whose origins, dynamics, and fallout may indeed have become unconscious. In this way, we hoped to explore what was going on in the communities in conflict and how the emotional legacy of The Troubles—and the transgenerational transmission of trauma—were manifesting themselves currently.

Large-Group Identity

The emotional legacy of The Troubles, built on the longer history of oppression and conflict between the UK and Ireland, over time, became embedded in large-group identity. This is an extremely important concept. As most clearly developed by Volkan (2020), large-group identity has to do with common, often highly charged identity elements held by thousands, even millions, of people who will never meet each other. Rooted in generational history, they provide a secure and continuing answer to the question, "Who are we?" Those answers may have to do with race, religion, nationality, some combination of these, or some other large-scale group designation. Large-group identity is not a conscious process and does not begin in the late adolescent phase of identity formation—crucial as that phase is to the individual's further identifying with, or differentiating from, the large group.

Rather, large-group identity is an emotional phenomenon beginning in early life, with a child's earliest identifications, and continuing during the phase when a toddler is, both excitedly and fearfully, experimenting with leaving the home base of mother to explore a brand-new world. In the course of this, the child quickly takes in messages of "Here, with me, is safe. There is dangerous." And "here" generalizes from mother to family to home to village to religion to nationality. It also generalizes from safety to pride and morality. Things that belong "here" are good. Things that belong "there" are dirty or bad.

Beginning as a kind of collective stranger anxiety, large-group identity involves deeply internalized meanings related to one's own group, of sameness, safety, goodness, pride, and belonging, and meanings related to those outside the group, of otherness, shamefulness, and potential danger. If a group's anxiety is low, those meanings about the other may include less problematic emotions, like curiosity and generosity. But if a group's anxiety is high, latent meanings of the other group as alien, threatening, or dirty may become prominent, and at critical moments, a process of societal regression can be set in motion.

In the Little Museum of Dublin, there is a framed statement by the singer Bono:

> The American looks at the guy with the big house on the hill and says, "I'm going to be that guy someday." The Irishman looks at the guy with the big house on the hill and says, "I'm going to get that guy someday."

A stereotype to be sure, but its kernel of truth speaks to gut-level large-group identity, shaped by colonization and trauma over centuries.

Bullets Through Time

"Bullets don't just travel through skin and bone. They travel through time." This statement was tattooed onto the shoulder of a young woman whose father was shot during The Troubles. It captures the emotional legacy of trauma, the way that the next generation and even subsequent generations must deal with what happened to people they loved and are deeply connected to. Sometimes this transmission leads to further violence, sometimes to mourning and reparative efforts. One way or the other, it's on the skin, so to speak; it's an inescapable part of a person's emotional life.

In Northern Ireland, real resolution of emotional difficulties has been difficult to achieve. There is considerable suspicion and a resigned weariness about reconciliation efforts. Some participants in the Corrymeela meeting wondered if this set of conversations would be genuinely useful or, as one participant put it on the first day of the gathering, if they were "just going around in the cement mixer again." But, from a psychoanalytic perspective, spontaneous metaphors may be revealing at a deeper level. "Going around in the cement mixer" seems fruitless, but it also prevents a dangerous hardening. The metaphor raises a question about this sort of peacemaking effort: Whether or not a given intervention proves valuable, is the continued work preventive in itself? Does it at least keep things in motion and some measure of hope alive? Of course, repeated disappointment can lead to profound skepticism and withdrawal from the work. The fact that so many people came to Corrymeela suggested cautious but ongoing hope.

The Hand

The day before the retreat began, my IDI colleague Dr. Robi Friedman arrived and brought a small gift to the member of our team who had initiated the project, Lord John Alderdice. A citizen of Northern Ireland himself, Lord Alderdice was deeply involved in the peace process for years (Alderdice, 2010) and, when the Good Friday Agreement was finally negotiated, he was elected the first Speaker of the Assembly. The gift was a porcelain hand making a sign of peace.

That evening, Dr. Friedman and I encountered a different hand. As the sun was setting, we walked down the hill from Corrymeela, along the coast and into the small town, where we visited a pub. We sat at the bar, ordered our pints, and chatted about the upcoming meeting. The atmosphere was jovial on the surface but edgy underneath. A man seemed to be singing loudly into his friend's ear. The young woman behind the bar looked at her regulars with resigned exasperation.

Then a young man—perhaps in his 30s—sitting next to my colleague abruptly introduced himself, welcomed us to the pub, and asked where we were from. He seemed completely drunk, an impression confirmed by his garrulous speech and by his repeatedly thrusting his hand toward us for handshakes over the next half hour. We were taken aback not just by his raucous intrusion but by the fact that all of the fingers on his right hand had been cut off at the knuckle. This man seemed to have been the victim of an industrial accident. He was both very friendly to us but also very angry, and he seemed to want us to see, from a psychoanalytic angle, his castrated hand. As we walked back to Corrymeela, my friend and I felt we had encountered something profoundly painful in Northern Ireland's current culture.

The Observers

In the formal meetings of the retreat, four members of the IDI facilitating team sat in a large circle with enough chairs for the other 21 invited participants. A fifth IDI facilitator sat with the small ecumenical group outside the circle. They remained silent during the discussions, taking up an observer role, perhaps representing, psychologically speaking, the Northern Ireland public in general. We had asked the ecumenical group to participate as observers because the methodology they have used in similar dialogues was quite different from ours, and we felt the mix of methodologies would not be a good fit. We were thinking psychodynamically, listening to personal stories and feelings, paying attention to defenses, working with group dynamics, and focusing on understanding the psychological obstacles to dialogue. We were not appealing to reason nor to morality nor trying to solve a particular problem. Our belief is that members can solve problems far better than us *if* they can really talk.

But we also wanted the ecumenical group to participate in some role. They had invited us; they were our hosts, and they wanted to learn about different forms of dialogue. So, after each session, the IDI facilitator met with them separately, collected their impressions about what they had observed, and helped them understand the interventions of the facilitating team. The IDI facilitators also met privately after the sessions, evaluating what they had observed and learned, listening to reports of the observers' views, and making decisions about how to proceed during the next session. At the end of the last session, a summary of the facilitators' findings and the observers' perceptions were shared with everyone in the room for general discussion.

Leadership

The decision about the ecumenical group was one of many we as the leaders of the retreat had to make, and, of course, leadership issues came into the process as well. As the first meeting was about to begin, we learned that one participant had had to drop out and another would be arriving late. Thus, there were two empty chairs in the large circle as we began, which happened to be the two chairs on either side of the lead facilitator, Dr. Volkan. This may seem like a strange coincidence, but, from a psychoanalytic perspective, when people enter a group—especially an emotionally charged one—they pay subtle attention to where they sit.

What did it mean that no one sat next to the lead facilitator? One hypothesis would be that he represented authority, perhaps authority attributed to him as an accomplished person, but also the authority of someone who represented the risky task they were about to take up. Indeed, there may well have been some fear in the group's reactions to Dr. Volkan. Perhaps also, in such a bitterly contested larger environment, no one may have wanted to be seen as trying to curry favor with the person in authority by sitting next to him.

But this potential pairing dynamic—that is, the wish to gain advantage by forming a power couple with the person in authority—seemed present in an informal moment just before the session began. This moment too involved a hand. A young charismatic politician from one of the Nationalist parties—a party that wants Northern Ireland to unite with the larger Republic of Ireland—reached out to shake hands with Dr. Volkan and said, "Welcome to Ireland!" not "Welcome to Northern Ireland." The struggle to have the person representing authority on one side and not the other seemed to have begun.

Looking for a Third

In fact, the desperate search for a leader was the first major theme of the conversation. In various ways, people communicated an intense need for someone who had the power to contain and tame aggression, someone or something that could function as a stabilizing third structure. First, participants turned to the police officers in the group. When the senior police representatives tried to explain logically how the

Northern Ireland police institution worked—that it could not serve a partisan purpose, nor, in an effort to manage such widespread aggression, turn the society into a police state—disappointment ensued. The officers felt caught in the middle in this group, as they also felt themselves to be in the society.

Then the participants searched for other symbolic leaders, such as religious institutions and even business organizations. The clergy in the room at times attempted to fill this role, sometimes movingly, other times with frustration. One clergyman's story of how he called on his community to reclaim their church square from militants was a concrete and, it turned out, successful example of a citizen's effort to claim the societal space. Then a business leader pleaded that the economy and education were crucial issues that could bridge divides, if only groups could get past their rage. Finally, someone petitioned for a "bill of rights." The facilitators spoke to the participants' preoccupation with finding a stabilizing "leader," an institution, an overarching cause, in psychoanalytic terms, a "shared superego" to help contain frightening, potentially destructive feelings.

Since the overall population was fragmented, no one leader in Northern Ireland was currently able to accomplish that stability. Of course, aggression in civic life is necessary, in the form of raising one's voice, asserting a right, and demanding recognition. But, sadly, in Northern Ireland, aggression had for years been expressed primarily as violence, and, even after the Good Friday Agreement, it still was. No leader had been able to help this traumatized large group restore its basic trust in each other and in a way of living together.

Dr. Volkan's leadership was exercised primarily in the management of the event. Sessions started and ended on time. Dr. Volkan set out the task at the beginning, invited people to speak openly and personally about their problematic experiences, and asked the group for a critical authorization. "I ask you, with all due respect, to allow me to say, 'Shut up!' if I feel someone is giving a speech," he said. This elicited laughter and easy consent from the group, but it was extremely important to the group's confidence that, at least in the microcosm of the retreat, someone would indeed manage aggression. And, managing it made it possible to talk about it specifically and directly. Another important intervention early on was Dr. Volkan's question to a man who reported having been in jail for a considerable period of time. "What were you in jail for?" Dr. Volkan asked. "Murder," the man said, in front of police officers, though he added that, from his point of view, he was a soldier who had killed in combat.

Shame and Community

During the initial session, the women—none of whom were politicians—were completely silent. Northern Ireland has been a patriarchal culture, at least at the political and leadership levels, for a very long time. When we noted the women's silence in this first session, the group realized that almost all of the nonpolitical leadership—men and women—had been silent. They seemed to be living out one person's idea that they were "spare parts." Again, an interesting metaphor; "spare parts" conveys a sense of being useless but, in fact, spare parts are essential when something breaks down.

On the other hand, the politician members of the group—all men—spoke easily, although in ways that sounded at first like party platforms. This could be understood as their way of grounding themselves in their political identities and establishing security at the beginning of an anxiety-arousing discussion. But it was not a dialogue across representatives of different groups nor was it personal. The team noted that real dialogue across the political/nonpolitical boundary was difficult, and so for a while the conversation was in a state, as one member put it, of "suspended animation," just as the politics of Northern Ireland were.

When this was noticed and understood, women among the participants found their voices and spoke about the feelings they were holding. One set of feelings erupted in response to a story one of the clergy members told, a poignant story about having bought a new tie for a family celebration. Then, walking down the street, he was greeted by one of his parishioners with a bitter question about whether he was ashamed to wear his collar. That question may well have related to the sexual abuse scandal in the Catholic Church, but, in the moment, it left him shocked and deeply hurt. Quite strikingly, the group did not pick up at all on the obvious pain this man had brought to the conversation. It was as though nothing had happened.

When a facilitator noted this and referred to shame as a potential psychological obstacle, another member burst into a rage: "How dare you speak about shame?" Then she added, "Don't you know that there is so much shame in all of us that if we allowed ourselves to feel it, we would all kill ourselves?" This almost primal outburst highlighted two emotional obstacles to the group's and perhaps the community's moving forward. First, to speak the feelings made them real. It was as though the facilitator had not simply heard what the clergyman had just said about shame; he had made it real by speaking it. In this sense, he had inflicted it on the group. Second, having become real, the shame was now dangerous to the very community essential to getting through these terrible feelings. "We would all kill ourselves" is a profound statement that the community-in-the-mind simply would not survive the intense feelings of its members. These participants seemed to be saying that there was no holding environment for them, no collective capacity to contain together the shame of actions done to each other over so many years. Hence the longing for some third party outside the community to serve this function.

Betrayal

Other intolerable feelings eventually came into the conversation: guilt for abandoning past injustices; wishes for retribution intermixed with, and sometimes identified with, demands for justice; and existential fear of the other group. To some degree, the emotional engagement around shame—brought into the work by one of the women members—seemed to free people, especially among the nonpolitical subgroup, to join the discussion. The political leadership, however, seemed more invested, and perhaps more stuck, in their positions. Was this the result of how powerfully they were carrying their constituencies' pain, grievances, and difficulty grieving? Ironically, the phrase "political class" was used a number of times, a phrase that could suggest being "above" the people. But did this distract all of us from how embedded political leadership is in the most basic and stubborn feelings of the people? Is this one reason that it can be difficult to exercise real leadership in the face of constituents' resistance?

This brought into the discussion the question of loyalty to one's group. Real feelings of loyalty to one's group intermixed with fear of being seen as disloyal and seemed to bind members of the same group together, both in the meeting and in the society as well. As one member put it, "I'm part of a group that will be suspicious of you, so I'm morally bound to be suspicious." And, more frighteningly, should one be or appear to be disloyal, "the danger is from our own group." The history of The Troubles is full of lethal punishment for real or suspected disloyalty, and the words of an Irish poet are a rule to live by: "Whatever you say, say nothing."

This question of loyalty presents an enormous problem for political leaders, who are elected by a part of the community but must lead the whole community. In the context of violent rivalries, there is a major risk—to electability and to safety—in being seen as betraying one's own group. But real leadership sometimes requires what a colleague calls "virtuous betrayal" (Krantz, 2006), that is, a leader's taking decisions that may betray a narrow, emotional, and even self-defeating interest of a constituency in favor of a greater, encompassing good. One politician described how his bipartisan work on the damage sectarian fighting had done to children's education was met with a grandmother's rage. "How dare you talk with the people who killed my grandson," she said. "My dilemma," he said to the group, "is I betray the past or I betray the future."

Grievance and Grief

This grandmother's pain captures the distinction between grievance and grief. The legacy of The Troubles is full of deep grievances that, at a psychological level, function as a powerful defense against grief. Grievance looks toward a future in which revenge of some sort or at least some compensatory righting of a grievous wrong will occur. Grief, on the other hand, is about a loss that is now in the past. Whatever has been lost, usually a person, is irrecoverable. In one sense, there is no future certainly for the lost loved one but also as it is felt by those grief-struck individuals left behind. The only real way forward is through mourning. But the trauma of sudden loss makes opening up the mourning process very difficult, especially for those who have suffered so many losses over so long a time.

As the sessions proceeded, we began to hear more personal stories, which were very moving. Because the group had begun to work with each other and with us, and because time was short, Dr. Volkan made a critical intervention:

> I am sure that most of you in this room and perhaps all of you experienced losses during The Troubles. You lost family members, friends, things that you deeply value. Psychologically, it is necessary that after important losses, people mourn. People die, things disappear, but their images, their "mental doubles" remain in our minds. We have an internal relationship with these mental doubles, which goes on until we say goodbye to them over time, until they become futureless, so to speak. If everything goes well, such internal relationships slowly come to rest. But, in Northern Ireland, such losses were linked to severe traumas and conflicts. So, my hunch is that such mental doubles are still very much around. What do they tell you?

Initially there was anger about this intervention because it invited participants to open up very difficult emotions. At least two participants stated they were not there "to be psychoanalyzed." They even suggested that the facilitator needed their permission before making this statement. Clearly, a frightening question had entered people's thoughts; if the community might kill itself because of shame, how could it survive the unbearable grief built up over so many years? Soon, however, the dynamics changed when one member dared to speak his own mind. "Are you kidding?" he said to the more resistant group members. "Ghosts are everywhere in Northern Ireland!"

Following this, participants began to talk about lost friends and relatives, and about what those "ghosts" were telling them, so to speak. They began to realize that, without going through and dealing with their complicated grief reactions, unspoken feelings remained alive in the mourner. At a group level, being stuck in a shared but warded-off mourning process forces traumatized communities to unconsciously hold on to other problematic emotions: survival guilt, wishes for revenge, shame for being friendly with the opposite side, guilt for abandoning past injustices, an unending list of grievances, and confusion about how to deal with victims. This discussion showed that even rational people must deal with "ghosts." Without the presence of a stabilizing "leader," this group (representing Northern Ireland's various communities) seemed to need outsiders (the facilitators) to help open and care for these "wounds." Now they were beginning to see how the intensity and pervasiveness of traumatic loss had become a profound emotional obstacle to peacemaking.

Another Hand

One of the Nationalist leaders repeatedly stated how his party was extending its open hand to political opponents so that everyone could "move forward" but that that gesture was always rejected. The facilitators noted that representatives of the Unionist parties—who want Northern Ireland to remain a part of the United Kingdom—were suspicious of these overtures. They felt that Nationalists had not really renounced their strategy, which the Unionists viewed as an existential threat, but had simply changed their tactics. Nationalists might give lip service to the reconciliation process but not really engage with it. The Nationalist side seemed unable to understand or alter this part of the dialogue. To them, the Unionists in the group seemed split among their own different parties, unclear about their stance, silenced by their own colleagues, and not ready to meet the offer of an "open hand."

Did this stalemate represent what was happening with the majority of the silent electorate, who might themselves feel culturally and politically disempowered? Were Unionists worried about simply surviving, in contrast to the main Nationalist party's sense that it was thriving? Were they worried about feeling abandoned by the British government, or something else? We did not have time to fully understand all of these issues. Nationalists did not seem curious about their opponents' refusal to join them and did not present their own genuine arguments for societal change. Nor was empathy for the other's experiences a part of the culture of communication between these groups; it was as though empathy risked betrayal of one's own side and humiliation by the other. Meanwhile, "The Hand" once again emerged as a metaphor for working toward peace or refusing it.

In this context, Lord Alderdice found himself thinking about the mythic origins of Northern Ireland, and he brought to the group's attention the meaning of the Irish symbol, the Red Hand. According to mythology, the North had no rightful owner and was claimed by the two most powerful clans in the South. The clans' leaders agreed to a race between the fastest runner from each clan; whoever's hand first touched the land of the North would be its owner. As the two runners neared their goal, one saw that he was about to lose and so cut off his hand and threw it ahead onto the soil of the North. Thus, a claim was made and the battle started. The bloody "Red Hand of Ulster" is actually a ubiquitous symbol in Northern Ireland and emerged in the discussion as a powerful metaphor, capturing a deep, life-or-death sense of rivalry between two warring groups. The story being told in this moment, not only of rivalry but of bad faith agreements, felt like a powerful intervention. An important historical and cultural context—a Genesis story really—had been discovered, one that cast grave doubts on what it means to work together.

The myth of the Red Hand of Ulster brought to our attention another "hidden" emotional factor that most likely plays a role in preventing a settling of The Troubles in Northern Ireland: a stubbornly enduring, conscious and unconscious culture of rivalry, which stirs the adrenaline even if its actual goals are mythic and its means of achieving them unfair. After the Corrymeela meeting, we learned more about how the symbol of the Red Hand is very much "alive" in Northern Ireland. It is part of the provincial and political flags of Ulster and Northern Ireland. Its image is deployed frequently by the Ulster Volunteer Force and other loyalist paramilitaries (including the Red Hand Commandos). The Gaelic Athletic Association uses it for one of its county teams. A Red Hand marks burial plots maintained by the National Graves Association, adorns stained-glass windows in Belfast's City Hall, and even advertises the services of Indian palmists.

For decades, the Red Hand was the logo for the Northern Ireland Tourist Board, though it has since been replaced by a heart. As I have noted elsewhere (Fromm, 2022), people sometimes put right there on the mantelpiece, so to speak, a critical signifier of their trouble. Hidden in plain sight, it becomes unconscious to them, but available to others, as though inviting an interpretation of, to mix metaphors, the water the fish is swimming in and can't know for itself. Adam Phillips (1996) notes that psychoanalysis is about secrets that one can only tell oneself by telling someone else.

Respect

In the final session, a young Unionist, who to that point had been the only silent member of the group, said to a Nationalist: "You extend your hand, and say you want us to join you but, when we don't, you interpret that as our problem, rather than asking us *why* we don't join you." He was pointing out how real curiosity was missing from the Nationalist's approach, in favor of presumptions and defensive certainty. It was as though Nationalists felt they already knew the answers, so didn't need to ask the questions. Indeed, it was generally true for the entire group that inquiry into why someone felt a certain way or hesitated about joining was largely missing, as though to genuinely explore issues across this highly charged political boundary was dangerous.

The Unionist then added, referring to a comment made earlier in that session: "And why do you want us to respect your dead? I respect my own dead; I don't need you to respect them." Then, one of the Nationalist members—to that point a jovial, collaborative sort of person—spoke with genuine feeling:

> I'll tell you why. When I was growing up, people didn't even acknowledge that my mother and father and grandmother even existed, and when they did, they treated them like dirt. So, if they weren't respected in life, I want them respected in death.

An NGO leader, formerly a senior police officer, responded, in a way that joined with the facilitators: "That's what they mean by the *ghosts of the past*." Then he said to the Nationalist: "I won't remember much of the political talk here, but I will never forget what you just said."

Words that are unforgettable—unforgettable because so profoundly and personally true—are one of the most important outcomes of any intervention into trauma. In the relatively short time of the retreat, we noted a number of hopeful progressions. Over the course of the five sessions, there was increasing emotional engagement throughout the membership, an increasing capacity to tolerate the expression of feeling, and increasing strength in the voices of the civic leadership. Related to this, there was more person-to-person talk, including, very importantly, the political leaders' speaking personally. After phases of resistance, members joined the facilitating team's consultation and shared personal experiences of trauma and loss. Finally, new leadership emerged, along with important bridging issues and a number of hypotheses that might shed further light on the emotional dynamics of this conflicted but very appealing community.

Another Third

The IDI facilitating team left the retreat feeling very grateful to the participants for the risks they had taken and for their growing trust in our capacity to contain and make sense of the strong feelings they expressed. For various reasons, this was a one-time intervention, the outcomes of which, whatever they were, were carried back by individual members into their political and societal roles. We learned that there were some behind-the-scenes communications between a few participants that seemed to move in a constructive direction.

While it was probably being planned long before the retreat, the Centre for Democracy and Peace-Building (CDPB) was founded in Belfast not long after the retreat. Led by two of the retreat's participants, the CDPB institutionalizes the larger task, of which the retreat was a part. It tries to find "entry points" within Northern Ireland's political and social dynamics for actions that might diminish the power of the psychological obstacles that emerged in the retreat. In doing so, it works to counter community fragmentation and despair. Traumatized societies are seriously at risk of collapsing back into traumatizing conflict.

The CDPB is a concrete third space, as the retreat was a process version of that thirdness. This is one of the major contributions psychoanalysis can make to societal conflict: the building of third spaces in which potentially overwhelming feelings can be contained, made personal, and made sense of. As noted earlier, this takes psychoanalytic leadership to establish the analytic task and to manage the analytic frame. It then takes lending one's analytic responsiveness to the process that emerges. And it takes a commitment to neutrality—a sometimes embattled concept these days—through which one can listen empathically and nonjudgmentally to both sides. In dialogues between enemy groups, neutrality is essential because the minute one side feels that the other side is favored, the dialogue is over.

We, as the retreat's facilitators, did not know how this group's problems should be solved, and we didn't make suggestions in that direction. Rather, we trusted the unfolding process and trusted that, with a good enough process, the members themselves could come to solutions. This too is a form of respect. It is a testament to the Good Friday Agreement and to the perseverance of people, like those who organized and participated in the Corrymeela retreat, that so far this battered, tenacious, and profoundly alive group of people is still working hard to solve its own problems and to build a thriving community.

Note

1 Portions of this chapter expand on material previously published in the following works:

From "On the mantelpiece: Organizational trauma in plain sight" (Chapter 6) in Traveling through time: How trauma plays itself out in families, organizations, and society, by M. G. Fromm, 2022, Phoenix Publishing House. Copyright 2022 by Phoenix Publishing House. Reprinted with the kind permission of the publisher.

From Chapter 17 in We don't speak of fear: Large-group identity, societal conflict and collective trauma, edited by V. Volkan, R. Scholz, & M. G. Fromm, 2023, Phoenix Publishing House. Copyright 2023 by Phoenix Publishing House. Reprinted with the kind permission of Karnac Books Limited.

References

Alderdice, J. (2010). Off the couch and round the conference table. In: A. Lemma & M. Patrick (Eds.), *Off the couch: Contemporary psychoanalytic applications* (pp. 1–15). Routledge.

Fromm, M. G. (2022). On the mantelpiece: Organizational trauma in plain sight. In *Traveling through time: How trauma plays itself out in families, organizations, and society* (pp. 73–93). Phoenix Publishing House.

Krantz, J. (2006). Leadership, betrayal and adaptation. *Human Relations*, *59*(2), 221–240.

Phillips, A. (1996). *Terrors and experts*. Harvard University Press.

Strozier, C. (2025). *Making peace in Northern Ireland: The miracle of the Good Friday Agreement and the creation of a fair and just democracy*. Ethics International Press.

Volkan, V. (2020). *Large group psychology: Racism, societal division, narcissistic leaders and who are we now*. Phoenix Publishing House.

Volkan, V., Scholz, R., & Fromm, M. G. (Eds.). (2023). *We don't speak of fear: Large-group identity, societal conflict and collective trauma*. Phoenix Publishing House.

Chapter 5

Writing Matrescence

Therapeutic Writing Retreats as Collective Containers for Transgenerational Healing

Tracy Sidesinger

Literary writing is a deeply psychoanalytic process. It allows individuals to open up to their conflicts, follow a path of free association, interact with multiple self-states through editing, and form a reflective, coherent narrative. In particular, small group therapeutic writing retreats focused on matrescence help women going through the long transition to motherhood to use these psychoanalytic principles at a crucial developmental period and in community with others.

Maternal experience became the focus of these writing retreats to counterbalance the limited attention such experience receives in psychoanalysis and in much of society (Sidesinger, 2024a). There is a documented tendency to show more interest—in both literature (Daly & Reddy, 1991) and psychoanalysis (Grill, 2019)—in what it is like *to be mothered* rather than to be or become a mother, even when an individual has both experiences. This dissociative gap in our collective understanding has profound impacts on intrapsychic, interpersonal, and collective registers. Psychoanalysis has historically viewed pre-Oedipal states as "regressive" (for example, Mahler, 1960), thereby inscribing such states with a pejorative or even pathological nature, without sufficient consideration for what these states mean for the adult mother equally taken by them. In doing so, psychoanalysis abandons mothers on their journey of parental development and inadvertently nurtures in them a mother wound.

Furthermore, a proliferation of social ideas about motherhood and "good parenting," when received in a formulaic approach, may influence mothers to repress thoughts and feelings that don't comply with social expectations and therefore diminish their reflective functioning. This represents a subtle but insidious collective harm. Absent space for

DOI: 10.4324/9781003658382-6

their own voices, mothers can be disconnected from personal subjectivity, intersubjective care, and maternal knowing, the consequences of which alter the collective.

At the same time, matrescence brings with it a sense of urgency. It highlights the importance of mentalizing so as not to reproduce problematic patterns of behavior and attachment styles and instead recognize and support a child's individuality within a family system. Following on Winnicott (1953) and others, Rundel (2022) has begun to elaborate on "unitive states, first experienced in early life, not as pathological, but rather as the crucible for passionate relationship and creative vitality" (p. 472). It is in this spirit of encouraging mothers to access creative vitality, reflective yet close to the source, that these retreats were conducted.

Additionally, teaching mothers how to develop a reflective writing practice helps to address some of the accessibility issues of psychoanalysis for this population. While even the most reflective writing practice is not equivalent to psychoanalysis, it will be shown that there are significant parallel effects of both methods. Advantages of writing include that it can be done at any spontaneously available time around caring for young children and that it is more cost-effective than psychoanalysis, a concern for mothers who usually do not get financially compensated for their care labor.

Theoretical Base for Matrescence Writing Retreats

Writing as Method

The initial basis for offering writing retreats as a form of applied psychoanalysis lies in the established value of writing for therapeutic purposes. James Pennebaker and his student Sandra Beall (1986) began studying expressive writing after his earlier health research revealed that people who experienced abuse and kept it secret were most likely to have various health problems. He hypothesized that opening up about trauma would help to reduce symptoms, but he was also aware that telling vulnerable secrets to others could be a liability. Writing thus was a way to speak one's experience, regardless of the presence or absence of a safe other to whom one could tell it. In subsequent years, Pennebaker's (2018) research on expressive writing has demonstrated that it is associated with a long-term reduction in symptoms, helping individuals work through trauma as well as form identity through narrative structure.

Pennebaker's expressive writing and a number of other therapies incorporate writing into therapy, though many of these tend to utilize a cognitive-behavioral orientation, guiding participants toward desired outcomes such as promoting forgiveness, wisdom, and gratitude and focusing on thoughts (Ruini & Mortara, 2021). While these are certainly useful techniques, writing can also parallel psychoanalytic processes and be used to support the emergence and working through of unconscious contents. In her musings on life writing in aging women, Hanscombe (2018), a relational psychotherapist and memoirist, also suggests that writing is an analytic endeavor. Halton-Hernandez (2020) similarly notes how Marion Milner encouraged the exploratory creativity of her patients and herself through writing. Milner experienced writing as a means to foster "continuity of being" in ways that the couch—owing to its dyadic dependencies—could not facilitate in the same way (p. 243). Writing allows the writer to give voice to what has been kept secret and to create coherence and meaning through what is necessarily an active, personally driven process.

Literary writing—such as memoir, creative nonfiction, and the essay—has particular affinities with the psychoanalytic approach. In her introduction to *The Best American Essays*, Leslie Jamison (2017) explicated the meaning of the verb "essay": it is to try, to make an often tentative or experimental effort to perform. The essay, to Jamison, "investigates its own seams. It traces what leaks" (p. xviii). Yet in order to succeed, essays also have to be focused so as to generate insight by way of nuance. She continued,

> If essays aren't immune from failure, they *are* singularly equipped to metabolize their own failures, to follow the smoke signals of these failures toward better versions of themselves, to take what might feel like an obstacle—shame, confusion, contradiction, muddled memory—and confess it, investigate it, probe it.
>
> (p. xviii)

Thus essaying can be an act of writing the questions into some form of narrative coherence, but through a meandering, unsettled, and free-associative approach. The essayist does not set out with a linear argument to prove. Rather, she is driven by conflict, a multifaceted question in search of formulation, and through this pursuit she becomes her own witness.

Writing into Psychic Conflict

Unconscious conflict is the meat of psychoanalytic discourse, and in her book *Torn in Two*, Parker (2005/1995) argued for the reality of conflict to be restored to our modern understanding of motherhood:

> The suffering of ambivalence can promote thought—and the capacity to think about the baby and child is arguably the single most important aspect of mothering. Perhaps this becomes clearer if we invent a hypothetical mother who does not experience ambivalence but regards her child only with hostile feelings, or conversely only with untroubled love. In neither case will she find it necessary to dwell on her relationship with her child or to focus her feelings on her child's response to herself because she will not know what is missing. It is the troubling co-existence of love and hate that propels a mother into thinking about what goes on between herself and her child.
>
> (p. 9)

Parker goes on to say that wrestling through ambivalence is what leads to "expanded consciousness." By free associating on the page, leaving and then returning in another state, whether to write again or come back as one's own editor, multiple self-states present themselves in a visible tension. This is akin to how Bromberg (1996) conceived of psychoanalysis as a relational environment in which individuals can come into contact with the "normal multiplicity of the self." He saw the mind "as a configuration of shifting, nonlinear, discontinuous states of consciousness" (p. 516) and sought to help individuals experience different aspects of themselves, deepen awareness of their coexistence, and bring them into conversation with one another. Dobrich (2020) has brought particular attention to dissociated states in "motherless daughters" who are thus engaging in identity in terms of lineage and the fraught ambivalence that can subsequently accompany mothering. The application of relational dissociation theory has thus been shown to be appropriate to working with mothers.

Editing in particular supports the recognition of a person's multiplicity and ambivalence. Feelings are contradicted, words are unintentionally repeated, and things that made sense in one's head don't make sense on the page. Amidst all this, the editorial self must find a way to bring such discrepancies into sufficient narrative cohesion to pass as a unified self or to represent the fractures of a subject struggling to integrate.

Writing to Develop Mentalization, a Position of Thirdness

Practiced in a manner of free associating and reassociating what has been dissassociated, literary writing serves as a form of mentalization and creating "thirdness." In such a state one is able to take perspective, reflecting on their motives and meanings, as well as their impact on others. Literary writing here is differentiated from journaling, which—while helpful as a means of being with one's internal mind and affective states to begin with—may not engage relationship to the outside world, conflict, editing, and revision. These latter tools in particular align with the conditions necessary for the creation of thirdness.

Reflection, also referred to as "mentalization" (Bateman & Fonagy, 2013), is a key component of a psychological mindset. According to Bateman and Fonagy, mentalization is "a profoundly social phenomenon," what others might call intersubjective, working to remember that others have internal minds as well and are not simply objects in one's own world (p. 595). This goes hand in hand with one's capacity to "think" and not just enact patterns of behavior.

I find it helpful to consult other theorists on how one develops the capacity to think, and here Britton's (1989) case comes to mind in which he reported being told to "[s]top that fucking thinking!" (p. 88). He understood this as the patient's response to perceived threat in the parental couple—as if consulting one's own mind was a form of inner intercourse mimicking parental intercourse. Thus, Britton (2004) conceived of thirdness through the "triangular space" between two parents and a child—"the possibility of being a participant in a relationship and observed by a third person as well as being an observer of a relationship between two people" (p. 46). Benjamin (2004) considers thirdness with maternal subjectivity in mind and argues that thirdness does not originate as a paternal function. Even from the beginning of a child's life, mother and baby are already distinct. Preverbally, the mother holds the tension in her observing mind between the baby's distress and her own empathy. The "third in the one," Benjamin writes, is "analogous to the ability to project the child's future development (in other words, her independence)" (p. 12).

In Benjamin's conceptualization, the third is inherently relational. It cannot exclude the actual other or exist exclusively in the realm of thought. Herein lies the heart of intersubjectivity and relational psychoanalysis. On some level, then, reflection cannot be done without another, even when it is done in one's own mind. A more pointed statement would be: one's capacity for reflection is intimately connected to their capacity for relating.

Writing for Matrescence

Matrescence itself is a tumultuous process for individuals going through it. According to the definition by Athan and Reel (2015), matrescence is a significant change across all dimensions of life:

> Much like adolescence, but nested in the niche of mid-life, it is an experience of dis-orientation and re-orientation marked by an acceleration of changes in multiple domains: physical (changes in body, hormonal fluctuations); psychological (e.g., identity, personality, defensive structure, self-esteem); social (e.g., re-evaluation of friendships, forgiveness of loved ones, gains in social status, or loss of professional status), and spiritual (e.g., existential questioning, re-commitment to faith, increased religious/spiritual practices).
>
> (p. 9)

Not only is matrescence a time of upheaval, disorganization, and reorganization, but it has also been co-opted from mothers to mean something abstract, general, and one-sided, serving patriarchy more than mothers or children. In her recent, widely popular book *Matrescence*, Jones (2023) described why she found it necessary to write such a book. "I started to realize that my mind had been colonized by inadequate ideas about womanhood, about motherhood, about value, even love. There was canker in the roots of my habitat" (pp. 9–10). Thus where most attention during this time has gone to the new child, mothers' psychological processes also need attended to—and in fact more so during this developmental period as compared with other, less transitional times in their lives.

But as Benjamin (2004) pointed out, we are already in maternal territory when considering reflective capacities. For a mother to take time to reflect on her own experience already requires thinking about the other. The mother must have some capacity for both identification with and separateness from the child in order for them to both go on being. Dobrich (2022) described using a patient's birth story to help them understand internalized, inchoate images of themselves and working toward verbalized expression of the meaning this birth narrative held for his mother as distinct from his own sense of self. Turning the tables, we also consider here what can happen when mothers are supported in narrating the stories of their children's births (among other things) through a lens of thirdness, long before the child grows to adulthood.

In fact, mothers are one population with whom mentalization-based treatment has been applied and found effective. Bate, Bekar, and Blom (2018) summarized existing data that mothers with insecure attachment styles tended to show a lack of narrative coherence as well as an increase in avoidance of distressing or unresolved attachment experiences. Furthermore, when mothers are able to think about their own experiences, they are less likely to reenact behaviors that lie at the heart of non-secure attachment styles (Fonagy & Target, 2005; Slade et al., 2005). On this basis Steele and Steele (2008) posited that "a central aim of intervention and prevention work must be to encourage reflective functioning in parents or parents-to-be" (p. 133). Simultaneous to a process of differentiating between a mother's own experience and that of her child, she may also reflect on the interconnected aspects of their co-created lineage (Sidesinger, 2023, 2024b).

Writing in a Group Context

Lastly, groups were thought to be the most appropriate context for extra-analytic writing retreats. Goodman and Santangelo (2011) found evidence across studies that group therapy is effective for reducing distress and treating postpartum depression, perhaps because they act on the isolation that so many mothers experience. Additionally, where all families keep secrets in one form or another, nonfamily groups that nonetheless discuss familial dynamics evoke these issues in a more verbal, consciousness-raising way. In her elaboration of meta-dialogue, Dobrich (2020) considered that group work offers a "unique contribution … in transforming dissociatively enacted self-states associated with early object loss into an enlivening meta-dialogic process within intersubjective and intrapsychic realms" (p. 368). Groups support multiple dimensions of reflection by pointing to the universality and deep interconnectedness of experience and making more visible what is otherwise dissociated.

Again, taking a perspective that reflection is not a function of paternal thought that imposes separateness but actually of connectedness, the type of reflection that these writing retreats supported is also unitive. Rundel (2022) elaborated on "unitive" as contrasted with "regressive" states through the lens of psychedelics. Psychedelic experience—much like matrescence—points to

> united states beyond the personal unconscious, toward a felt sense of connection with all beings and all of reality, a transpersonal layer of consciousness …. It also offers a way to start to think about the ancestral healing that is often a part of psychedelic experience.
>
> (p. 473)

As already indicated, matrescent epistemology

> can consider the child-in-the-present as different from the parent, yet related in their origins, part of an ongoing relationship to their specific lineage. When a mother can differentiate her child from her own child self, the underlying relation between them does not disappear, but can become more clear.
>
> (Sidesinger, 2024b, p. 97)

Thus, groups underscore that even individually produced writing operates through relationality and is inherently directed toward it.

The Therapeutic Writing Retreat Experience

Application Process and Participants

Participants discovered the writing retreats through social media, therapists, and other word-of-mouth recommendations. Retreats were advertised as women's-only weekend group experiences "to submerge in ancestral deep time." Specifically, it was stated that writing prompts and group sessions would be used, facilitated by a seasoned psychotherapist and author. Before applying, potential participants were prompted to think of these retreats as therapeutic, group-based, and focused on writing as the primary method of consciousness-raising around transgenerational issues at the site of motherhood.

A typical advertisement included the following preamble in everyday, accessible language:

> The page, before it is anything else, is our witness. But by this I mean not only journaling but also writing with skill and craft. That's because living a psychological life means taking on your story as your own. Yes, it may begin with a simple transcription of events, but a psychological life always requires facing the hard stuff, letting go of the story you thought you knew, and creating the story that is only yours to tell. Writing is the place where we confront our own voices most profoundly.

Interested individuals were required to submit a free-form application describing why they felt drawn to the retreat and how it fit into their current writing lives. This was useful for orienting individuals toward reflective writing even before the retreats, beginning in their usual environments and preparing them for a more intensive period of writing. Participants also had 30-minute one-on-one orientation calls with the facilitator beforehand, as is common practice in facilitating groups. These calls further clarified the use of group process and personal editing as tools to support more insight into the issues each person was bringing to the retreat.

Some individuals expressed interest in participating but were unable to attend due to financial constraints or lack of childcare. Scholarship funds were established to support greater access to attendance for low-income and unpartnered parents and ensure a plethora of positionalities would be manifest in the group. Application and attendance were nonetheless skewed toward White, cisgendered, and partnered women, suggesting that access to resources still had some impact on who was able to gain from this extra-analytic offering. Future psychoanalytic writing courses will take this into consideration in order to further increase access, perhaps adopting a multi-week workshop format over that of intensive weekend retreats. Even for those who were unable to attend, the prospect of such an opportunity seems to have had an impact on helping mothers recognize that reflection on their identity, behavior patterns, and family planning is even an option.

One participant described in her application her projections onto the retreat as an anchor for preserving her own identity, which was otherwise hard to come by:

> Since I first came across your retreat on Instagram in September, I haven't stopped thinking about it. Every time my toddlers rip a pen from my hands as I try to list out the reasons for my anxiety, I think of this retreat. Each time my husband calls, "Mommmyyyy!" from another room, I think about this retreat. When I sit down to write and notice how my belly now rests in my lap—a reminder of the changes two back-to-back pregnancies during a pandemic have made to my body—I think about this retreat. Every time I am surrounded by students calling me "Mom" and bombarded with questions, I think about how badly I need this.
>
> (Applicant, Personal Communication, 2024)

Another applicant, an established writer, sought out interpersonal space where she could deepen an existing focus on her role in intergenerational issues:

> Having been a mother myself for five years, I'm finding myself wanting to shine a light on my own identity as a mother, separate from my identity as my mother's child. I believe I need a roadmap for how to move into the future as a mother and I want to write this roadmap myself.
>
> (Applicant, Personal Communication, 2024)

This participant described her prior experience writing motherhood as painful and isolated. She was interested in having a group context in which to support her writing where she felt blockages.

A first-time mother of a six-month old simply wrote, “I’ve been wanting to write more about my birth experience to help process and make sense of it. It’s been hard to find the space/time.”

Applicants had diverse reproductive identities and, for those who identified as mothers, had children in a range of ages from six months to those preparing to graduate high school. It was widely recognized—both by the facilitator and participants—that though the perinatal period is a peak moment of matrescence, maternal identity is constantly shifting and in need of ongoing attentive reflection. Some were actively choosing not to have children but sought out space to consider their decision in relation to their maternal lineage and other relationships.

Furthermore, the experiences represented by participants were a diverse and rich tapestry. They included perinatal mood and anxiety disorders such as depression, anxiety, OCD, and PTSD, but were approached by each individual with a sense of narrative agency, as participants understood the retreat was not a treatment setting. As such, symptoms were reflected on within the broader landscape of social and family systems and, more so, cohesive personal identity. Some concerns that participants addressed included pregnancy loss, anger at the medical system, and anxiety about future pregnancies; facing internalized parental neglect and compensatory overextension as a mother; and reckoning with what did and didn’t happen during the child’s developmental years.

Writing Retreat Structure

The retreats took place at a home in Upstate New York. Onsite, participants could gather for group sessions, write independently, eat together, walk in nature, and sleep overnight. Retreats began with a happy hour to meet others and share intentions while getting comfortable in their shared space. An hourly schedule was given beforehand, including planned silent time, as well as four interactive group sessions.

Group sessions consisted of various activities designed to foster interpersonal engagement and generate writing material. Sessions varied and morphed based on the needs of each group. The opening session always consisted of each participant sharing a photograph of their mother and an object that represented their intentions for the retreat. Participants spent time during the session writing as an objective observer about the photograph they shared. This exercise helped participants alter perspective on their mothers and contrast it with their affective, subjective experiences. They were invited to share portions of their writing with one another and enter the retreat with a sense of lineage as well as conflict (along the lines of Parker, 2005/1995, referenced earlier).

Subsequent sessions utilized model texts to explore participants' feelings around different aspects of their lineage and maternal experience. These included but were not limited to excerpts from *Matrescence* (2023) by Lucy Jones; *All Fours* (2024) by Miranda July; *What My Mother and I Don't Talk About* (2019), an anthology edited by Michele Filgate; and *On Earth We're Briefly Gorgeous* (2019) by Ocean Vuong.

Vuong's (2019) autofiction is written to his mother after her death, laden with his sexuality, an embodied story impeccably rendered in relation to the body of his mother. He writes of their experience as immigrants from Vietnam to the United States, which serves also as a cultural subtext for the abuse he experienced at the hand of his mother. As such, *On Earth We're Briefly Gorgeous* is a text of literary conflict: Vuong's mother is not an "all good" or "all bad" object, but one to whom the author relates with complex honesty and an inseparable identity. Vuong also writes about writing, even in his fiction. Toward the end of this novel, he acknowledges that there is always the possibility of continuing the family lineage, fated and unchanged, "falling off the cliff like buffaloes," but there is also the possibility of intercepting the family narrative through writing. "Ash hardened to ink on a blank page," Vuong writes, "the story that turned 'shrapnel' into 'art'" (p. 233). Though Vuong doesn't have or write about his own children, his experience of his mother is instructive for lineage writing. His sense of coming into sexuality in particular embraces the conflict of both identifying with and differentiating from mother.

Similarly, as part of the anthology *What My Father and I Don't Talk About* (2025), Julie Buntin explores the transformations of self- and family-narratives over time, most especially during matrescence. She writes,

> There's another version [of my childhood], a secret I keep to myself as a child, watering it until it grows: I am a forgotten girl. I believe in that version long past childhood. Until one day, when I am thirty-three and pregnant with my first child. My father sends me an email, and the story transforms again.
>
> (p. 266)

These and other texts helped prompt participants to consider the impact their writing could have on their lives, and home in on topics of personal resonance.

Group sessions also employed activities aimed at drawing out "hot spots" in each participant's family lineage. These included drawing life timelines, mapping family trees, and imaging family constellations (following Manne, 2009) through the use of neutral objects. In mapping family trees, for example, participants were asked to include as many people as they could remember and then color in the hot spots, such as who died young, who was forgotten, is anyone estranged? Participants might be asked questions, such as Where is there significant emotion? Do you notice where there are patterns of close bonds? Are any other patterns apparent? Is there a particular energy that seems to be absent in your family tree?

These intertextual, experiential groups thus focused on hot spots, patterns, and relationships, stirring up topics that each person could then explore through free-associative writing. Some sessions involved sharing what had been written, while participants also had ample time to write independently. In coming back together with others who were similarly exploratory and vulnerable, participants tended to be receptive to feedback. At times, the group offered support to those expressing distressing or isolating experiences in their content. At other times, group feedback made note of themes that a writer herself might not have noticed or areas that seemed more unclear or unprocessed than a writer realized. For example, one participant observed that her uncle was surprisingly prominent in her birth story only when she shared it with the group. This allowed her to give voice to how her experience and that of her child felt unimportant in comparison to other members of her family. Feedback like this was then taken by participants into subsequent writing sessions where they could deepen their reflection on emotionally charged dynamics.

The group format also demonstrated the reality of co-created experience, where certain themes emerged as more prominent in each group. In one group, where all participants had young children, babies, or traumatic births, birth stories became an emphasis. In another group, participants noticed through the sharing of family trees that alcohol addiction was a common theme. These identifications allowed participants to feel validated in exploring their concerns. Furthermore, writing independently in addition to group process supported the development of agency and personal working through for participants.

Conclusion

Motherhood is a realm of fraught sociopolitical attention, which, in turn, demands attention at the collective level. As I write this, so-called anti-natalists pit themselves against pro-natalists, and abortion and fertility treatments are increasingly targets in the crosshairs of American politicians. These are of course but a few examples. There are many social forces that still compel mothers—in the enduring words of Adrienne Rich (1976)—toward lifeless "institution" more than "experience." At the same time, motherhood as experience is ineradicable. It is deeply personal, subjective, and continues to change over time. This clash between motherhood defined by external demands or internal processes need not be so binary. Instead, psychoanalysis could play an important role in creating space for mothers to speak in their own voices rather than being spoken for, and emerge as a collective subject.

"Large group identities," as conceived by Volkan (2014), are identities a person accepts for themselves yet which are derived from the groups to which they belong. Nationality and religion are two main examples. Volkan emphasized ways in which groups rise to significance relative to a sense of threat, reinforce tribalism, and can justify inhumane treatment of the Other by means of exclusionary identity. His work is immensely important for conceiving of psychological development and identity with regard to the collective. Yet, Volkan's definition doesn't account for the positive aspects of large group identity, such as a sense of origin, or the healthier dimensions of belonging to a community that fosters coherence and carries a shared cultural narrative.

Motherhood can be helpfully assumed as a large group identity insofar as it is personally accepted and articulated but also experienced within a register of communal belonging. Psychoanalytically informed group experiences like the matrescent writing retreats described here do just that. They simultaneously help individual subjectivity to emerge in resistance to imposed narratives, while repairing and reimagining what it means to belong to the universal group of mothers.

References

Athan, A., & Reel, H. L. (2015). Maternal psychology: Reflections on the 20th anniversary of *Deconstructing developmental psychology*. *Feminism & Psychology*, *25*(3), 311–325.

Bate, J., Bekar, O., & Blom, I. (2018). A mother, a baby, and two treatment approaches: Discussing a switch case from CBT and mentalization perspectives. *Journal of Infant, Child, and Adolescent Psychotherapy*, *17*(4), 328–345. https://doi.org/10.1080/15289168.2018.1526159

Bateman, A., & Fonagy, P. (2013). Mentalization-based treatment. *Psychoanalytic Inquiry*, *33*(6), 595–613. https://doi.org/10.1080/07351690.2013.835170

Benjamin, J. (2004). Beyond doer and done to: An intersubjective view of thirdness. *Psychoanalytic Quarterly*, *73*(1): 5–46. https://doi.org/10.1002/j.2167-4086.2004.tb00151.x

Britton, R. (1989). The missing link: Parental sexuality in the Oedipus complex. In J. Steiner (Ed.), *The Oedipus complex today: Clinical implications*. Karnac.

Britton, R. (2004). Subjectivity, objectivity, and triangular space. *The Psychoanalytic Quarterly*, *73*(1): 47–61. https://doi.org/10.1002/j.2167-4086.2004.tb00152.x

Bromberg, P. M. (1996). Standing in the spaces: The multiplicity of self and the psychoanalytic relationship. *Contemporary Psychoanalysis*, *32*(4), 509–535. https://doi.org/10.1080/00107530.1996.10746334

Buntin, J. (2025). I was so hopeful for you. In M. Filgate (Ed.), *What my father and I don't talk about: Sixteen writers break the silence* (pp. 265–292). Simon & Schuster.

Daly, B. O., & Reddy, M. T. (1991). *Narrating mothers: Theorizing maternal subjectivities*. University of Tennessee Press.

Dobrich, J. (2020). An elegy for motherless daughters: Dissociation, multiplicity, and mourning. *Psychoanalytic Perspectives*, *17*(3), 366–384. https://doi.org/10.1080/1551806X.2020.1801053

Dobrich, J. (2022). The creative use of birth stories in psychoanalytic treatments. *Psychoanalytic Social Work*, *29*(2), 109–122. https://doi.org/10.1080/15228878.2022.2086437

Filgate, M. (Ed.) (2019). *What my mother and I don't talk about: Fifteen writers break the silence*. Simon & Schuster.

Fonagy, P., & Target, M. (2005). Bridging the transmission gap: An end to an important mystery of attachment research? *Attachment & Human Development*, *7*(3), 333–343. https://doi.org/10.1080/14616730500269278

Goodman, J. H., & Santangelo, G. (2011). Group treatment for postpartum depression: A systematic review. *Archives of Women's Mental Health, 14*(4), 277–293. https://doi.org/10.1007/s00737-011-0225-3

Grill, H. (2019). What women want: A discussion of "Childless". *Psychoanalytic Dialogues, 29*(1), 59–68. https://doi.org/10.1080/10481885.2018.1560867

Halton-Hernandez, E. (2020). The Milner method: Marion Milner and Alison Bechdel's autobiographical cures. *Life Writing, 18*(2), 243–260. https://doi.org/10.1080/14484528.2020.1717912

Hanscombe, E. (2018). Now that I'm old: Life writing, women and ageing. *Life Writing, 16*(1), 127–138. https://doi.org/10.1080/14484528.2019.1521645

Jamison, L. (2017). Introduction. In L. Jamison & R. Atwan (Eds.), *Best American Essays 2017* (pp. xvi–xxvi). Best American Paper.

Jones, L. (2023). *Matrescence: On the metamorphosis of pregnancy, childbirth, and motherhood.* Allen Lane, Penguin Random House UK.

July, M. (2024). *All fours.* Riverhead.

Mahler, M. S. (1960). Symposium on psychotic object relationships—III. Perceptual dedifferentiation and psychotic 'object relationship'. *International Journal of Psychoanalysis, 41*, 548–553.

Manne, J. (2009). *Family constellations: A practical guide to uncovering the origins of family conflict.* North Atlantic.

Parker, R. (2005). *Torn in two: The experience of maternal ambivalence.* Virago. (Original work published 1995)

Pennebaker, J. W. (2018). Expressive writing in psychological science. *Perspectives on Psychological Science, 13*(2), 226–229.

Pennebaker, J. W., & Beall, S. K. (1986). Confronting a traumatic event: Toward an understanding of inhibition and disease. *Journal of Abnormal Psychology, 95*(3), 274–281. https://doi.org/10.1037/0021-843X.95.3.274

Rich, A. (1976). *Of woman born: Motherhood as experience and institution.* W. W. Norton.

Ruini, C., & Mortara, C. C. (2021). Writing technique across psychotherapies—From traditional expressive writing to new positive psychology interventions: A narrative review. *Journal of Contemporary Psychotherapy, 52*(1), 23–34. https://doi.org/10.1007/s10879-021-09520-9

Rundel, M. (2022). Psychedelic psychoanalysis: Transformations of the self. *Psychoanalytic Dialogues, 32*(5), 469–483. https://doi.org/10.1080/10481885.2022.2106139

Sidesinger, T. (2023). Reproductive agency and the transgenerational transmission of trauma. *Contemporary Psychoanalysis, 59*(1–2), 64–85. https://doi.org/10.1080/00107530.2023.2242578

Sidesinger, T. (2024a). Introduction to the special issue on maternal subjectivity: An essential link in relational-social psychoanalysis. *Psychoanalytic Perspectives, 21*(3), 281–305. https://doi.org/10.1080/1551806X.2024.2377936

Sidesinger, T. (2024b). Maternal excess: Pathways through overwhelm to transformation in the perinatal period. *Studies in Gender and Sexuality, 25*(2), 93–103. https://doi.org/10.1080/15240657.2024.2346455

Slade, A., Grienenberger, J., Bernbach, E., Levy, D., & Locker, A. (2005). Maternal reflective functioning, attachment, and the transmission gap: A preliminary study. *Attachment & Human Development*, *7*(3), 283–298. https://doi.org/10.1080/14616730500245880

Steele, H., & Steele, M. (2008). On the origins of reflective functioning. In F. N. Busch (Ed.), *Mentalization: Theoretical considerations, research findings, and clinical implications* (pp. 133–158). Analytic Press.

Volkan, V. D. (2014). *Psychoanalysis, international relations, and diplomacy: A sourcebook on large-group psychology*. Routledge

Vuong, O. (2019). *On Earth we're briefly gorgeous*. Penguin.

Winnicott, D. W. (1953). Transitional objects and transitional phenomena. *International Journal of Psycho-Analysis*, *34*, 89–97.

Chapter 6

Confronting the American Gun Complex

A Jungian Analysis of Mass Shootings

Randi Gross Nathenson

Columbine, Pulse Nightclub, Tree of Life Congregation, and Uvalde are names that are now indelibly engraved upon the American psyche, eternally linked to incidents of mass shootings. These words elicit profound feelings of grief, horror, and helplessness. They signify not only the tragic loss of life and the devastating injuries but also deep wounds in the collective soul of the nation. Despite this profound scar, there has been little substantive action in response to these tragedies.

Each time a mass shooting occurs, one wonders whether this will finally serve as the tipping point, the moment when Americans collectively declare, "enough," and demand action. In the interim, the aftermath of each mass shooting has yielded an eerily predictable response. Expressions of thoughts and prayers, attribution of blame, debates on gun control, and finger-pointing ensue, followed by an unsettling silence. The silence reflects a national dissociation of sorts, a space where the outrage dulls into quiet resignation. The overwhelming feelings of grief and terror are numbed and made tolerable. In this collective disempowerment, mass shootings are viewed as routine occurrences rather than tragic anomalies.

Instead of action, there is a tendency toward finger-pointing; we seek to understand the motive, the rationale, and the circumstances surrounding the event. In hindsight, the events leading up to the tragedy are reconstructed. Various pieces align in a jigsaw-like manner as we search for signs and indicators. We endeavor to make sense of the senseless. This cycle repeats itself, seemingly without resolution or transformation. The energy generated following each tragedy swiftly fades, sinking into the unconscious and remaining unprocessed. But the grievance of chronic mass murder remains there just below the surface until the next time it erupts.

DOI: 10.4324/9781003658382-7

Amid the finger-pointing after each mass shooting, few ask the harder or deeper questions, and there is little to no thorough reflection. Gun control advocates blame guns, violent video games, and bullies, whereas gun rights advocates blame the parents and loosening moral values. Both sides strive to find a sufficient scapegoat on which to project their personal and collective shadow.[1] The assumption is that finding the cause means solving the problem. This quick-solution cause-and-effect thinking is emblematic of American culture, which focuses on symptom eradication rather than the telos. What is ignored is our own violent nature, in essence, the would-be mass shooter in each of us, our disowned rage and aggression. What remains unaddressed is the symbolic nature of the gun, one which is central to our cultural identity, which tends to be either literalized or discarded entirely rather than integrated into our collective understanding.

Gun violence is rooted in the archetypal dimensions of American history and culture. At the heart of this lies the American gun complex[2]—a profound, largely unconscious psychological entanglement. Operating across personal, cultural, and archetypal levels, it weaves together identity, collective mythology, and weighty emotional undercurrents. A deeper understanding of the gun's cultural significance is essential to grasping the complex's grip on the collective psyche. This complex shapes our personal and cultural identities and fuels resistance to meaningful change, impeding efforts to address root causes and implement real solutions.

Like the Stars and Stripes or apple pie, the gun has become an emblem of being American, carrying a sacred, almost religious significance. Its symbolism is intertwined with the constitutional right to bear arms and national ideals such as freedom, opportunity, and independence. Mass shootings expose the destructive force of this complex and the danger in treating the gun as a sacred object. Each mass shooting represents not just an isolated tragedy but an archetypal possession: a constellation of the gun complex overtaking the ego, where unintegrated elements of power, rage, and aggression are expressed with fatal consequences. In these tragedies, cultural and personal dimensions converge, exposing the shadow side of America's relationship with guns.

Mass shootings are statistically rare, accounting for 0.1% of all homicides (Duwe, 2004). Despite this, they permeate our collective psyche more than other, more common forms of gun violence. Mass shootings are not a unique phenomenon to the United States; however, what is unique is the rate of mass shootings, our response to them, and our gun culture. In "Public Mass Shooters and Firearms: A Cross-National Study of 171 Countries," Adam Lankford (2016) explored the assertion that mass shootings are a primarily American problem by completing a study that examined incidents in 171 countries from 1966 to 2012. Lankford found that the United States had the largest number of mass shootings by far, with only four other countries (the Philippines, Russia, Yemen, and France) reaching the double digits.

What further distinguishes the response to mass shootings in other countries is the adopted approach. In her article "How Australia and Britain Tackled Gun Violence," Margaret Hartman (2015) examined the reactions to mass shootings in Australia and Great Britain, underscoring their divergent perspectives in comparison to those in the United States. For instance, on March 13, 1996, in Scotland, Thomas Hamilton legally acquired four handguns and tragically took the lives of 16 children along with their teacher at an elementary school. Hartman indicated that subsequent to the massacre, the Parliament enacted the Firearms Amendment Act, which prohibited certain firearms and imposed restrictions on the sale of firearms at gun shows. This was followed by additional legislation that effectively contributed to gun violence mitigation.

The United States has a unique gun culture that differentiates us from other countries, adding complexity and nuance to the conversation. The birth of our nation was archetypal—a rebellion against tyranny. This shaped our identity; as a nation, we felt required to act in self-defense. Guns were significant in the formation of the United States, helping us to win the Revolutionary War, granting us the power to massacre Native Americans, and aiding in the expansion of our conquered territory under the ideology of manifest destiny (Hofstadter, 1970). Guns remain an icon, an archetypal image of the country that has become concretized to embody what is sacred to Americans: individualism, freedom, rights, and power.

While the gun functions as a symbol of national independence, it equally represents the capacity to conquer and dominate the original inhabitants of the land. In the United States, where a coherent and inclusive national identity was initially absent, the gun served as a compensatory object, offering a fantasy of self-sufficiency, hypermasculine independence, and impenetrability. Yet this fantasy was not only defensive; it also enacted a deeper historical script, one in which power is asserted through violence, and identity is secured through the subjugation and erasure of others.

Robert Jay Lifton has argued that American gun culture is different than that of other countries because we lack a traditional base:

> America was built on patterns of movement around the constantly moving frontier and continuous immigration. We also didn't start with a traditional culture in place; maybe no country does, but we had even less of one to begin with. So in America we have all sorts of cultures coming together and forming the concept of "the American." But our *identity* has always been shaky, and we've always been uneasy about our lack of a longer history and of a traditional culture. Sometimes that uneasiness has made us emphasize what history we do have all the more strongly. So what I'm saying is that as a country we tend to look for ways to compensate for the absence of a traditional cultural base. And in my view the identity we've built around conquering the wilderness, the gun, and our constitutional right to self-defense together form a major compensation for that absence of tradition.
>
> (As cited in Peay, 2015)

If our origin myth centers around the gun, then we are going to hold the gun as sacred and resist its removal from its pedestal. Limiting access to guns in any way is therefore viewed as un-American. Many gun rights advocates argue that any infringement upon gun rights is an encroachment on our very existence, our way of being us. Threatening the complex threatens our very identity. The gun represents a fantasy of control and self-sufficiency in the American psyche in place of a secure, relational sense of self and community.

Jungian analyst Dennis Merritt (2013) points to American culture as primitive and regressed, a culture in which we have taken up arms to solve our problems: "This is where America is stuck: we have not gone beyond the adolescent mentality of the conquering phase of our myth of the West with its guns to the mature, civilized, law-and-order phase" (para. 5).

Guns are connected to the American dream, which is focused on achievement, success, autonomy, and material desires. While many contemporary Americans reject this mythology and seek alternative narratives grounded in justice and inclusion, others continue to cling to it consciously or unconsciously as a way of maintaining a sense of identity rooted in dominance, rather than mutual recognition. Symbolically, the American dream reinforces the cultural ethos of manifest destiny and westward movement, of settling the frontier, and the gun provides us with the means to do so and a potential solution when we cannot. The gun has allowed those who have felt disempowered to engage with an archetypal symbol of power, to project power and death. Merritt explored how this archetype tends to be black and white; it divides things into good and evil, an either/or stance, which is supported in movies and television. As a result, we carry the image of the gun-toting cowboy, the myth of the American West, and the idea of rugged individualism that supports this conquering mentality. The inability to fulfill what is dictated by the American dream can lead one to feel like a failure, disempowered, full of shame, and worthless.

One of the commonalities among mass shooters is a deep sense of ostracization, inferiority, and disempowerment—a feeling of being cut off from their own agency and place in the world. In *Psychoanalytic and Spiritual Perspectives on Terrorism*, Nina Cerfolio (2023) explores the psychological profile of mass shooters through a psychoanalytic lens, highlighting how such individuals often experience profound internal fragmentation and unmet needs for recognition, belonging, and meaning. Their violent acts can be seen, in part, as distorted attempts to reclaim a sense of control or visibility—an effort to assert a fractured self in a society they perceive as having rejected or erased them.

These feelings and experiences are common, not just to mass shooters but also to many analysands who enter my consulting room. It is common for individuals to come to analysis questioning their lives, paths, power, and purpose. Underneath these emotions are anger or rage, feelings of being unvalued and disempowered, especially among those who lack ties to subcultures that provide counternarratives or other forms of expression and belonging. Notably, a significant number of mass shooters in the United States have been White, American, Christian, heterosexual men—individuals with the highest degree of privilege in American culture. For those raised within a framework that assumes entitlement to control, success, or social status, the experience of failure, rejection, or insignificance can feel especially intolerable. When life doesn't match the internalized promise of privilege, it can provoke a crisis—not just of identity, but of moral order. If you've been told, explicitly or implicitly, that the world is supposed to recognize and reward your existence, the lack of that affirmation can be experienced not just as disappointment, but as a personal affront. In this light, privilege can function like a psychic double-bind: it confers invisible advantages but also imposes silent demands. When those demands are unmet, and no language for healthy struggle is available, the resulting alienation can be both profound and dangerous. In extreme cases, that rage gets projected outward in violent and catastrophic ways.

In his essay "A Psychology of Bullets," (2000) Glen Slater explores gun violence as the shadow side of the cultural expectations of the American dream. Slater examines our obsession with the idea that everyone could (and should) rise up and become something, preferably wealthy and successful, valuing materialism above all else. Slater states, "Beneath the cloak of normative goals and aspirations, we have fervently embraced a cluster of social values that can be identified as precursors of gun violence" (p. 20). The inability to fulfill this dream constellates an affective experience, including a sense of rejection, alienation, and anger, necessitating a corrective response that can turn violent.

> The gun appears when the gap between actual life and the idealized American Dream opens too wide; the gun is fired when there is no *thing* left to satisfy the belief that we make our own destiny … the role of the gun is to extend and protect willful intent when self-image and personal goals are threatened.
>
> (p. 21)

In the absence of achievement, the gun becomes a validation.

In this context, it is understandable that the gun debate is emotional, affect-ridden, and extremely polarized, often along political party lines but also along racial lines. For many White Americans, especially those who identify with a narrative of rugged individualism and self-protection, gun ownership is tied to identity, freedom, and autonomy. For many communities of color, however—who have historically been subject to state violence and systemic neglect—the presence of guns often evokes vulnerability, surveillance, and danger. The "two sides" refuse to listen to each other or compromise, viewing the other as wrong. The gun debate creates a false dichotomy, an either/or mindset:

> The two groups compete with each other for political and social resources ... each of these groups considers itself part of the mainstream of the broader American culture while at the same time portraying the other as participating in a separate and irrational subculture.
>
> (Utter & True, 2000, p. 67)

The two sides do not listen to one another; instead, they engage in projection, perceiving the other as corrupt, imprudent, and irresponsible. This polarization ensures neither side hears the other. From the perspective of gun rights advocates, gun control advocates are seen as naive, dishonest, power-hungry, and irrationally afraid of guns. Conversely, the gun control side views gun rights advocates as paranoid, uneducated, regressive, power-hungry, dishonest about guns, and profit-hungry (Spitzer, 2012).

These supposedly diametrically opposed attitudes are part of the same cultural complex around the gun in America. There is little communication between these two groups because the beliefs within each culture are so strong, forming a complex in which these beliefs are deeply ingrained and in which the other side feels foreign and threatening to the potency of the complex.[3]

The gun is not just an object—it is a charged symbol, layered with meanings that extend far beyond its physical form. The symbolism of the gun is layered and multifaceted. The *Oxford English Dictionary* defines *gun* as "a weapon incorporating a metal tube from which bullets, shells, or other missiles are propelled by explosive force, typically making a loud, sharp noise" (n.d.). The etymology of the word *gun* comes from the Scandinavian Gunnhildr, meaning battle-maiden. Gunnhildr was a quasi-historical figure known for her cruelty and violence. Thus, the gun is personified, transformed from an inanimate yet deadly hunk of metal and plastic into a powerful, enlivened archetypal figure. This personification grants the gun a psychic life of its own, making it more than an object—it becomes a character in the American imagination, an actor in the cultural mythos.

The word *gun* is heavily interspersed throughout everyday language, in idioms and metaphors that represent power, rage, aggression, strength, impulsivity, speed, carelessness, and decisiveness, among other qualities. "Muscles" are referred to as guns, which people show off to display their physical power. The bigger a person's "guns" are, the more impressive they become because they symbolize strength, discipline, and power. A "hired gun" is a person who helps someone solve a problem or achieve power. When we talk about someone being a "son of a gun," they could be mean and unpleasant or someone tough who pulls through when needed. "Sticking to your guns" is about standing up for what you believe in and not swaying from that belief. A "smoking gun," though, refers to the decisive piece of evidence that proves someone's guilt. We call "shotgun!" when we want to sit in the passenger seat of a car.

We talk about the pressure of everyday life by saying we live "under the gun." We speak of "shooting for the moon" to encourage achieving our dreams. The phrase "gunning for your goals" suggests the process of trying to achieve something, with the gun providing the push to make it happen. However, someone who is "quick on the draw," "trigger happy," or "jumping the gun" or has an "itchy trigger finger" makes rash decisions or is careless or impulsive, which can have positive or negative connotations. We talk about "pulling the trigger" when decision-making is decisive. On the other side of this, being "gun shy" means you are tentative or afraid.

The gun is imbued with a multiplicity of paradoxical uses. It carries the capability of both life and death, survival and destruction. The gun can be used for hunting, protection, defense, and as a weapon of mass destruction. The gun becomes a vessel into which feelings of power, control, independence, and safety are poured, alongside deeper, shadow-laden drives: rage, domination, and death. For some, it is a sacred object of empowerment; for others, it is a symbol of fear and trauma. The gun functions as an equalizer and grants us power beyond our reach, regardless of physical size. The gun functions to arouse awe, reverence, and terror in equal measure.

This paradox is described in *The Book of Symbols* (2010):

> The gun plays an ambivalent role in the history of human survival and human carnage; hunting for food can be set alongside the extinction of entire animal species; the protection of home and hearth can be weighed against our staggering murder rates.
>
> (p. 498)

Guns touch upon a deep tension between the desire for safety and survival and the potential for rage and destruction. This tension highlights the shadow within the American gun complex, one that must be confronted and integrated, rather than split off and unconscious in order for meaningful change to emerge.

The gun is often seen as a phallic symbol, and the pleasure derived from shooting is frequently described as erotic. It connects the shooter to both generative and destructive instincts—power, sex, death, and life, all encapsulated in one seemingly simple device. There is an erotic element present in mass shootings, possibly a grandiose and perverted display of one's phallic power or an extreme compensation for feelings of powerlessness and rejection.

The Second Amendment has become an almost religious doctrine that supports the American gun complex, reinforcing the importance of guns in our culture (Waldman, 2014). Owning a gun is a right, and many gun rights advocates argue that any infringement on this right is an encroachment on our very existence and way of life. Threatening the complex jeopardizes our identity. It supersedes safety and prevention; upholding the Second Amendment becomes more important than ensuring our children are safe in their schools and homes. In her article "There's Something About Uvalde: American Patriarchy and the Slaughter of Innocents" (2024), Jungian analyst Carolyn Bates states, "There is no getting around the sense that, in the United States, certain lives seem cheap in contrast to the mission to protect the sacrosanct Second Amendment" (p. 228).

Within the complex, the strongest and loudest voice is the most extreme—the NRA. The NRA holds the power, both financially and politically, and has an aggressive and violent edge, an extremism that feels paranoid and split off. The rhetoric feels as if members of the NRA expect another American Revolution any minute, that they will again need to take up arms against a tyrannical government that threatens their freedoms. Somehow, any background check or waiting period becomes a threat, a slippery slope to a dictatorship, and the demise of individual liberty. The NRA lobbies hard and works at convincing gun owners that liberals are going to take away their guns.

The gun debate exemplifies how, while the United States values unity, not division, we are extremely polarized. Zoja states, "[T]his culture of unity at all costs has transformed itself into a one-sided negation of shadow, that is to say, of divisiveness or divisions which are an ordinary human reality" (2009, p. 14). Rather than allow for tension and splitting, we instead insist on being in agreement, which permits no space for reflection, conversation, debate, and discussion. Rather than engage and be curious, we instead try to convince the other to pay attention to what supports and reinforces our "side." The complex remains rigid and intractable. Zoja (2009) states, "If consciousness accepts only one aspect of a polarity the other aspect sets up a clamor in the unconscious until repression no longer works and there is some kind of explosion" (p. 14).

This hostile and regressed stance might be understood by recognizing America's relative youth and immaturity as a country. Our gun culture is regressed because American culture remains undeveloped. An undeveloped psyche can stand behind—or against—the gun as the solution to our problems. However, an undeveloped psyche can also lead to projection and unconscious identification, which "captures an immature ego more readily and for a normally growing ego, projection becomes a natural process along with occasional and hopefully only temporary identification with an ideology or cause" (Roy, 2004, p. 70).

This is a space where the political and the psychological become linked, where the gun's symbolic place in the American psyche holds enormous influence over politics. In our culture, without individual reflection, we have an overidentification with the gun and its collective meaning. To both personally and collectively individuate, we must separate our current identity from the past and be conscious of our heritage but not identify with it. Roy (2004) warned, "When identification with an archetype takes place, a normal ego loses its bearing, is overwhelmed, and may even face a psychotic breakdown" (p. 71). Our cultural identification with the gun as sacred casts a shadow through which mass shootings have become the extremely destructive way of assimilating that power.

These tragedies are an aspect of the explosion, the destructive nature of the complex, the dark side of holding the gun as a sacred and archetypal object. The shooting is a way of maintaining and adhering to one's power. When stuck in energy that supports and encourages taking up arms as a solution to problems, the mass shooting becomes a viable resolution, a way in which power can be reclaimed and one can assert oneself, be heard, and be seen. What gets projected outward is the need to destroy, to annihilate, in order to support the ego position. I wonder if what is happening *symbolically* in the mass shooting is that the shooter has become caught up in an enactment of the complex, possessed by the archetypal energy of the gun.

Mass shootings, however, cannot simply be reduced to the proliferation of guns or our gun culture. Nor can it be reduced to any of the other common scapegoats such as bullying, mental health, video games, or moral decline. The problem is larger and deeper:

> Violence is symptomatic of an underlying anguish that cannot be magically diagnosed and medicated away … such interventions serve to hide the oppressive social structures long in need of replacement and in doing so silence calls for lasting changes in actual lived conditions.
>
> (Chalquist, 2014, para. 3)

White males most frequently perpetrate mass shootings, but just as this is not simply an issue of guns, this is not merely an issue of White maleness. The reasons for this trend have more to do with socialization than physiology, a result of patriarchy, privilege, toxic masculinity, gender stereotypes, and racial bias. While aggression is encouraged and even rewarded in White males, in females, and particularly in females of color, along with non-White males, the expression of aggression and rage tends to be viewed pathologically, is judged more harshly, and is discouraged. The question is not exploring what is innate in White men but how our culture promotes this violence by them.

Recent mass shootings in Atlanta, Georgia; Charleston, South Carolina; and Pittsburgh, Pennsylvania, demonstrate the connection of mass shootings to racism, misogyny, homophobia, and anti-Semitism. This highlights the connection of the gun to the maintenance of oppressive power structures. The history of guns in America, as well as the history of gun control, is also a history that is inexorably linked with systematic racism and sexism. As a symbol of power, the gun has become caught up in the struggle to harness and maintain power, and who has access to that power typically has been controlled and decided by White men. Gun control laws have historically been enacted as ways to bar people of color from buying guns. This was, in fact, one of the original goals of the KKK (Winkler, 2013). In the 1970s, the NRA turned from being a nonpartisan group that supported gun control to the extremist right-wing organization it is today, in part, in response to the civil rights movement. Gun rights became a political rallying cry that could run counter to freedom marches as Burbick (2006) recounted, "Individual ownership of weapons became the foundation of freedom and as a result conveniently countered the collective nonviolent political language of civil rights" (p. 91).

On a personal level, the American gun complex reflects profound feelings of vulnerability, power, and identity. Guns often represent more than tools—they become extensions of oneself, providing a sense of control in a world perceived as uncertain or threatening. This complex intertwines with unspoken emotions like fear, anger, and rage that many individuals find difficult to acknowledge or express openly. Beneath the surface, guns serve as powerful cultural symbols that engage with archetypal themes. Recognizing this archetypal dimension is essential for understanding why the issue resonates deeply and proves resistant to simple solutions.

Hillman (2004) refers to the gun as a Hephaestion instrument that allows us to "hold the gods in our hand, carry death in your purse" (p. 124). He states that the gun is

> a fearful thing of beauty that holds Ares, Aphrodite, and Hephaistos all together in a fine piece of metalwork.... Human beings love their weapons, crafting them with the skill of Hephaistos, and the beauty of Aphrodite, for the purposes of Ares.
>
> (p. 124)

The gun becomes a container for archetypal energies, allowing us to possess this power, to become like gods ourselves, and to concretize the symbolic.

While other archetypal energies are at play, in the strategic planning of the shootings, in the amassing of arms needed, and so on, it is Ares who drew me in. The archetype of Ares is an image of life that is uncontained, destructive, chaotic, and violent. Although this brutal and caustic force can be found in other mythological figures, I was struck by the story. Ares is neither a proud warrior god, nor a vengeful authoritarian deity. Ares is depicted as the rejected child of Zeus and Hera. The name Ares comes from the Greek word for "ruin" or "curse." His epithets include killer of men, destroyer, and murderer. Ares does not have the revered all-powerful authority of Zeus, who throws thunderbolts at whoever crosses him, nor does he hold the wisdom and strategy of Athena on the battlefield. Ares is despised by most immortals and experiences frequent humiliation both on and off the battlefield. Ares is not so much the god of war as the personification of the horrors of it: he is father to Phobos and Deimos, fear and panic. Ares revels in the violence, driven not by motive or the picking of a side but by interest in annihilation. The violence of Ares is violence that comes from a dark, wounded place, a raging response to injustice, rejection, and isolation, violence for the sake of revenge whether the circumstances demand it or not. It is a desire to reclaim power he feels he has lost or never had.

In art, Ares is often depicted in full body armor, carrying a shield and spear. His home is located in the wild, barbarous land of Thrace; the psychological landscape of Ares is intolerable and primitive, a space that can feel affectively unbearable. I wonder if a mass shooting is both this repulsive space and the result of being situated psychologically within in it.

Ares is not a noun, but a verb, the action that occurs on the battlefield. Ares is the mass shooting, with the gun, the shooter can evoke the nature of Ares, the ability to wipe out dozens with a hunk of metal and plastic. The mass shooting becomes an extreme way to reclaim one's power, to make oneself known and infamous, reclaiming what they believe is owed to them. The mass shooter is archetypally possessed, caught in an inflated state. Pulling the trigger sweeps the shooter into a reality that transcends human potential and allows for revenge and retribution. The myth of Ares gets played out in destructive fashion. I reflect on the desperate search for a motive after a mass shooting, and how there often is not one. Ares does not need a motive; when Ares is constellated, there does not have to be a reason to fight, just a desire, and anything can justify the conflict.

Ares, known for being beautiful, figures often in stories of affairs, particularly with Aphrodite. While this pairing may seem paradoxical, it speaks to psychological balance and conscious integration of one's destructive capacity. Harmonia and Eros are born from this union, speaking to conscious integration and the creative potential of Ares rather than an identification with or revulsion to it.

In the *Idea of the Holy*, Rudolph Otto (1950) explored the experience of the numinous and referred to the feeling as the "*mysterium tremendum*," an overwhelmingly powerful experience. Otto states that this feeling had the potential to be wonderful, but it also "has wild and demonic forms and can sink to an almost grisly horror and shuddering" (p. 13). This speaks to the creative and destructive potential of Ares. When constellated, the image can pair with the love and beauty of Aphrodite or the wisdom of Athena, or it can unleash the horror of the mass shooting. It is a psychotic place where strangers become one's abusers, those you have to seek revenge against. There is a rush of adrenaline and, yes, joy in the idea of taking up a gun and shooting, causing destruction and chaos. It is a place of wanting to be heard and seen. It refuses to be silent; it is as loud as possible.

The gun debate creates a false dichotomy, an either/or mindset:

> The two groups compete with each other for political and social resources … each of these groups considers itself part of the mainstream of the broader American culture while at the same time portraying the other as participating in a separate and irrational subculture.
>
> (Utter & True, 2000, p. 67)

Gun control advocates think guns symbolize violence, male dominance, and aggression and that using them is acting out regressive infantile fantasies. Gun rights advocates believe guns symbolize order, manliness, self-sufficiency, and independence and that using guns affirms their relationship to nature and history. The truth is that guns symbolize all of those things, and we need to hold this in balance.

As I engaged with both sides of the debate during my work on this topic, I became more aware of the polarization on both sides. What emerged was not merely disagreement, but a defensive foreclosure of curiosity. The two sides refused to listen to one another or compromise, each side disavowing the other's position as wrong and dangerous. Rather than seeking understanding, advocates on both sides appeared caught in a dynamic of projective identification, wherein the other was cast as wholly wrong, and misguided, an unending ideological tug of war that stirred emotions. Whichever side one identifies with, there are high levels of reactivity. In relationship to the gun, Americans are obdurate.

While I expected to feel more at home with the gun control advocates, what surprised me was the reaction I encountered when I attempted to bring the conversation into deeper psychological terrain: When I raised the idea that unacknowledged shadow might be at play not just "out there" but within us, I was met with defensiveness by those advocating for gun control. The suggestion seemed to destabilize something fundamental; it challenged the ideological narrative that gun control advocates have, a disowning of one's own inner violence and locating it solely in the other. It is this attitude that has the danger to perpetuate polarization and paralyze any capacity for genuine social change. Without a willingness to confront our own shadow material, we remain caught in a cycle of moral reactivity, unable to metabolize the very emotions that fuel the conflict. Such a shift requires recognizing the presence of the shadow in all of us. Taking social responsibility seriously involves the difficult but necessary work of shadow integration, cultivating the ability to reflect on our own capacity for contradiction, aggression, and complexity. Only through this inner work can we begin to reduce collective polarization and support more honest and generative engagement across difference in advocacy work.

Our cultural complex around guns is also a personal one that plays out in our consulting rooms, rage, anger, and aggression often being experienced by analysands, who struggle with integrating the Ares energy, or what I term "the inner gun." These affects enter our consulting rooms often, many times unconsciously, defensively, complex-ridden, and unintegrated. At times, these energies are directed outward while other times, inward. Edinger (1984) described suicidal and homicidal tendencies as being opposite sides of the same experience of rejection and alienation, a rupture in the ego-self axis. A response can be rage, turned both inward and outward.

Conscious connection to this power, to our own aggression and rage, gives us access to our inner gun; in this way, we have agency and control over it; we can ensure we don't simply "go off" or explode like "loose cannons." There are times when we need access to this energy, to use our gun—our inner power—to protect ourselves or others from harm, to stand up for ourselves, or at times to complete tasks. The inner gun is symbolic for maintaining our sense of self, staying grounded in our center.

In his books *Human Aggression* (1995) and *Human Destructiveness* (1991), Anthony Storr explores the nature of aggression, supporting the claim that there are positive and negative features to aggression, that it is, in fact, instinctive and needed: "Aggression seems clearly linked with self-preservation, self-assertion, and self-affirmation" (1991, p. 7). Aggression is also connected to standing up for oneself and asserting one's identity. Aggression allows for intentionality; it can drive behavior in a situation in which there is conflict or competition. Having safe and conscious access to one's aggression requires a sense of one's worth.

Rage in and of itself is neither positive nor negative; it is what one does with the rage that can be problematic. When unmediated or unconscious, it has destructive potential. All of us must get in touch with our rage and find ways to channel it. Jan Weiner (1998) talks about rage as holding more intensity than anger; anger is more controlled, less fiery, whereas rage implies a level of being out of control. Rage is hot, elemental, primitive, unpredictable, dangerous, and connected to shame. According to Weiner (1998), anger is more related to the ego, as it has a cognitive component and is, to a point, controllable, whereas rage bypasses the ego and comes from the Self. Jung (1960) posited, "When we are beside ourselves with rage we are obviously no longer identical with ourselves but are possessed by a demon or spirit" (para. 6). Rage emerges when someone's security is threatened, when there are injuries to self-esteem or pride, or when someone feels ridiculed, humiliated, or ignored. Reacting with rage to these injuries can be a regulator, proof that you know you have worth, value, and integrity. It is saying that you cannot do this to me or treat me this way. Anger and rage can be adaptive in response to a threat.

It is when anger and rage are unchecked that they can have destructive negative impacts. The problem is "too much socially sanctioned self-suppression … [where] anger and resentment build over time into a morbidly murderous rage" (Diamond, 1996, p. 13). In these cases, "Our unresolved resentment, anger, and rage has turned violent, toxic, cancerous" (Diamond, 1996, p. 20). I believe, as Diamond has asserted, that "most of us have been culturally conditioned to suppress our rebellious anger and rage, taught that we have no right to be irate about our state, that we stoically ought not cry out against our often-outrageous fate" (p. 26).

Aggression and rage are potential reactions when people feel cut off from their power, their sense of agency, or their sense of value and belonging. When feeling powerless, the gun becomes a potential solution. The gun allows the shooter to take out what he or she perceives stands in the way. The gun reclaims it—just aim and fire—which is why "mass killers, unable to assert their power positively in the world, become … powerful victimizers as opposed to powerless victims" (Diamond, 1996, p. 13).

When rage is unconscious, it is dangerous and can result in individuals "venting their venomous hatred and rage on innocent bystanders" (Diamond, 1996, p. 27), as happens in a mass shooting. Recognizing and integrating aggression and rage are important parts of the individuation process in which we come to understand our potential for becoming the aggressor and find our connection to our own power. This shadow work is a crucial part of analytic work, and the inner gun can be seen as a symbol for the development of a conscious connection to aggression, rage, and power, which are necessary to hold in consciousness.

We must also work to develop a connection with our individual and collective shadow on both an individual and a community level. It is in this reflection on our own destructive capabilities that we can gain insight into mass shootings and a deeper consciousness of the phenomenon. This requires a conscious integration of the archetypal nature of the gun, rather than an identification with or revulsion to it. It is a process of looking inward, both individually and collectively, to engage with these parts of ourselves. It's through this type of reflection—acknowledging our own destructive potential that we begin to create space for healing and transformation. The consulting room serves as a container for reflective engagement with the personal and collective—not to pathologize but to humanize and integrate these energies consciously. It is in this work that the analyst can explore these as meaningful expressions of psyche rather than something to be suppressed or corrected. The work for the analyst and analysand is to confront their shadow material, to reflect on their own relationship to power, rage, and violence. In doing so, analysis becomes not only a space for personal healing but also a subtle act of cultural repair.

The analyst acts as a witness to the unconscious life of both the individual and culture, listening for what lies beneath. This type of listening involves a willingness to metabolize the unspoken tensions and emotional residues circulating the gun complex and to reflect them back in ways that hold complexity rather than reduce it. The consulting room offers a unique space in which there is the potential to soften polarization by honoring the deep emotional meanings in both the individual and collective.

Having access to these energies also allows us to access our creative instincts. Jung refers to the process of individuation as a creative process, requiring work and conscious energy. In a letter written in 1932, Jung wrote, "The best way for dealing with the unconscious is the creative way" (1973, p. 109). Creativity can act as a constructive way of making sense of the inner chaos, of integrating our rage, aggression, and desire for violence. Diamond (1996) referred to creativity as the "constructive utilization of the daimonic" (p. 256), which gives structure to the darkness and chaos. The positive potential of aggression, rage, and power is my own creativity, and then "anger and rage can be an enlivening, transformative, creative, even spiritual force" (Diamond, 1996, p. 13). As Jung (1966) has written, "the unsatisfied yearning of the artist reaches back to the primordial image in the unconscious which is best fitted to compensate for the inadequacy and one-sidedness of the present" (para. 130).

In *The Creation of Consciousness*, Edward Edinger (1984) argued that "the purpose of human life is the creation of consciousness" (p. 17). Edinger imagined the expansion of consciousness as a modern myth, a myth that connects us to the Self. The Self, as defined by Jung (1968), is "not only the center, but also the whole circumference which embraces both conscious and unconscious; it is the center of this totality, just as the ego is the center of consciousness" (para. 44). As we become conscious of who we are, of our inner figures, our shadow, and our complexes, and are able to relate to them in a more authentic, self-aware manner, these parts become integrated rather than split off in the unconscious. When these contents are unconscious, there is the possibility that we will act out; we might identify with our shadow and respond in ways that are not genuine and can be outright dangerous.

In *The Vision Seminars*, Jung (1976) posited, "We are like onions with many skins, and we have to peel ourselves again and again in order to get at the real core" (p. 821). It is through consciousness that we can be fully who we are rather than ruled by unconscious personal and cultural complexes and shadow material. Jung examined this shadow material in *Civilizations in Transition* (1964), where he wrote in depth about Germany following World War Two, using the Germanic god Woton, or Odin, to amplify the collective shadow material of Nazi Germany. In "The Fight with the Shadow," one of the essays collected in the volume, Jung discussed the destructive capacity of what lies dormant in the unconscious if shadow material is not made conscious and integrated. As I read Jung's words, "If such a compensatory move of the unconscious is not integrated into consciousness in an individual, it leads to neurosis or even to a psychosis, and the same would apply to a collectivity" (para. 448), I wondered if there was a parallel to mass shootings, with these events being a destructive enactment of archetypal shadow material carried by the collective. In other words, responses are exaggerated due to something being amiss in the conscious attitude. Jung (1964) writes,

> To confront a person with his own shadow is to show him his own light. Once he has experienced a few times what it is like to stand judgingly between the opposites, one begins to understand what is meant by the Self. Anyone who perceives his shadow and his light simultaneously sees himself from two sides and thus gets in the middle.
>
> (para. 872)

Meaningful response to mass shootings demands a dual approach: the inner work of confronting the psychic wounds and shadow material that underlie the violence, and the outer work of systemic and legislative reform. This calls for deep personal reflection on our own attitudes toward violence, power, and control, as well as cultural work that interrogates national myths that glorify domination and radical self-reliance at the expense of connection and vulnerability. On a collective level, this work should include public discourse, community dialogue, and educational spaces that help individuals recognize and explore the disowned aspects of our shared identity. As we confront and challenge the complex, we find the potential for growth and development. In facing it, we open the possibility for individuation—both within ourselves and in the soul of the culture.

Notes

1 In Jungian terms, the shadow refers to unconscious part of the personality that contains the aspects of ourselves we reject, disown, or fail to recognize.
2 A complex in Jungian terms is a cluster of unconscious thoughts, feelings, memories, and impulses organized around a common theme with an archetypal core.
3 Jungian complexes also serve an important role in attempting to establish psychological equilibrium. They form around emotionally charged experiences—especially those that the ego cannot fully assimilate—and act as autonomous subpersonalities within the psyche. Complexes strive to compensate for imbalances in the conscious attitude. In this way, a complex may emerge as a protective adaptation, seeking to preserve a sense of inner coherence or defend against psychic fragmentation.

References

Archive for Research in Archetypal Symbolism (ARAS). (2010). *The book of symbols: Reflections on archetypal images*. Taschen.

Bates, C. (2024). There's something about Uvalde: American patriarchy and the slaughter of innocents. *Journal of Analytical Psychology*, *69*(2), 227–245.

Burbick, J. (2006). *Gun show nation: Gun culture and American democracy*. New Press.

Cerfolio, N. E. (2023). *Psychoanalytic and spiritual perspectives on terrorism: Desire for destruction*. Routledge.

Chalquist, C. P. (2014, May 27). No man is an island: Recognizing gun violence as a cultural symptom. *Huffington Post*. http://www.huffingtonpost.com/craig-chalquist-phd/ucsb-shooting-cultural-violence_b_5394343.html

Diamond, S. A. (1996). *Anger, madness and the daimonic: The psychological genesis of violence, evil, and creativity*. State University of New York Press.

Duwe, G. (2004). The patterns and prevalence of mass murder in twentieth-century America. *Justice Quarterly*, *21*(4), 729–761.

Edinger, E. F. (1984). *The creation of consciousness*. Inner City Books.

Hartman, M. (2015, October 2). How Australia and Britain tackled gun violence. *New York Magazine*. http://nymag.com/daily/intelligencer/2015/10/how-australia-and-britain-tackled-gun-violence.html

Hillman, J. (2004). *A terrible love of war*. Penguin.

Hofstadter, R. (1970). America as a gun culture. *American Heritage*, *21*(6). http://www.americanheritage.com/content/america-gun-culture

Jung, C. G. (1960). *The structure and dynamics of the psyche* (Vol. 8, Collected Works). Princeton University Press.

Jung, C. G. (1964). *Civilization in transition* (Vol. 10, Collected Works). Princeton University Press.

Jung, C. G. (1966). *The spirit in man, art, and literature* (Vol. 15, Collected Works). Princeton University Press.

Jung, C. G. (1968). *Psychology and alchemy* (Vol. 12, Collected Works). Princeton University Press.

Jung, C. G. (1973). *Letters (Vol. 1: 1906–1950)*. Routledge.

Jung, C. G. (1976). *The vision seminars* (Vol. II). Spring Publications.

Lankford, A. (2016). Public mass shooters and firearms: A cross-national study of 171 countries. *Violence and Victims*, *31*(2), 187–199.

Merritt, D. (2013, July 19). Guns and the American psyche. *Jungian Ecopsychology*. http://www.jungianecopsychology.com/2013/07/guns-and-american-psyche-dennis-l.html

Otto, R. (1950). *The idea of the holy*. Oxford University Press.

Oxford English Dictionary. (n.d.). *Oxford University Press*. http://www.oed.com/

Peay, P. (2015, August 6). The gun, the bomb, and the wound that will not heal: An interview with Robert Jay Lifton. *Psychology Today*. https://www.psychologytoday.com/blog/america-the-couch/201508/the-gun-the-bomb-and-the-wound-will-not-heal

Roy, M. (2004). Religious archetype as cultural complex. In T. Singer & S. Kimbles (Eds.), *The cultural complex: Contemporary Jungian perspectives on psyche and society* (pp. 64–77). Routledge.

Slater, G. (2000). A psychology of bullets: Gun violence and the American dream. *The Salt Journal*, *2*(1), 19–24.

Spitzer, R. J. (2012). *The politics of gun control*. Routledge.

Storr, A. (1991). *Human destructiveness*. Grove Weidenfeld.

Storr, A. (1995). *Human aggression*. Penguin.

Utter, G. H., & True, J. L. (2000). The evolving gun culture in America. *The Journal of American Culture*, *23*(2), 67–79. https://doi.org/10.1111/j.1542-734X.2000.2302_67.x

Waldman, M. (2014). *The second amendment: A biography*. Simon & Schuster.
Weiner, J. (1998). Under the volcano: Varieties of anger and their transformation. *Journal of Analytical Psychology*, *43*, 493–508.
Winkler, A. (2013). *Gunfight: The battle over the right to bear arms in America*. W. W. Norton & Co.
Zoja, L. (2009). *Violence in history, culture, and psyche: Essays*. Spring Journal Books.

Chapter 7

Grievance, Grief, and Group Building in Community Psychoanalysis

Addressing the Needs of Asylum-Seeking Children and Students with Disabilities through Collaborative Consultation with Educators in a New York City Public School

Billie A. Pivnick

Contemporary cultural, political, economic, and climatic realities challenge psychoanalysts to continue to extend our scope beyond conventional clinical consulting. Contemporary theorists and practitioners now recognize the inevitable connections between the psychic and social—the mutually constitutive links among individual minds, groups, and culture—offering psychoanalysts new possibilities for our praxis (González, 2020; Hassinger & Pivnick, 2022; Hernandez-Tubert, 2011; Pivnick & Hassinger, 2022; Tubert-Oklander, 2014; Tubert-Oklander & Hernández-Tubert, 2021). Indeed, many psychoanalytic theorists and practitioners now envision a *social psychoanalysis* inspired by recent research that shows how (dissociated) historical cultural trauma and social pathologies (such as xenophobia, racism, misogyny, homo- and transphobia), as well as extreme economic inequalities, threaten the integrity and health of communities (c.f., Layton, 2020).

Community psychoanalysts work outside the consulting room and apply psychoanalytic theories and methods to the communities themselves (Altman, 2011; Bermudez, 2019; González & Peltz, 2021; Hassinger & Pivnick, 2022; Pivnick, 2021, 2017b; Pivnick & Hassinger, 2022; Pivnick & Hennes, 2014; Sklarew et al., 2004). Indeed, some psychoanalysts contend that Freud's predominant bequest to future generations of practitioners is in the ways he applied psychoanalysis to social and community issues, with his contributions to the treatment of mental illness taking a secondary role (Twemlow & Parens, 2006). Of particular importance is his thinking about human development and his

DOI: 10.4324/9781003658382-8

understanding of group psychology, which point to interventions that can improve individual and social health by harnessing forces of maturation to motivate growth and change while providing a map of how society and the individual inevitably influence each other.

Historical Foundations of Community Psychoanalysis: The Challenge of Inclusion and Exclusion

The first collected writings depicting "community psychoanalysis" were published by Neil Altman (2011) as *The Analyst in the Inner City* and by Sklarew, Twemlow, and Wilkinson (2004) as *Analysis in the Trenches: Streets, Schools, War Zones*. Together, these books documented how analysts actively practiced in nontraditional ways, detailing projects in schools and police stations, in political consultation, and in disaster, war, and racial trauma recovery. But early founders of the William Alanson White Institute (WAWI; i.e., Clara Thompson, Erich Fromm, David Rioch, Janet Rioch, Frieda Fromm-Reichman, and Harry Stack Sullivan) were already advocating inclusion of an interpersonal, cultural perspective in the years between the World Wars (Frie & Sauvayre, 2022; Sullivan, 1953/1968).

An important aspect of the historical break from Freudian orthodox tradition that led to the founding of WAWI was its emphasis on maturity, defined by Clara Thompson not as conformity to the culture but as "sufficient freedom from anxiety to be able to deviate from the culture when he finds it necessary to maintain his integrity of when he is convinced that the aims of culture are bad for man" (Green & Crowley, 1983, p. 1). In the '30s, Harry Stack Sullivan founded a new psychoanalytic journal, *Psychiatry: Journal of the Biology and Pathology of Interpersonal Relations*, that deviated from mainstream psychoanalysis by viewing the social and cultural as factors in mental health and in taking an interdisciplinary approach; he was practicing a form of community psychoanalysis (then called "fieldwork") in his participant-observation interviews of an interracial group of employees in the pantry of Walker Percy's home in Greenville, Mississippi (Stephens, 2022).

The analytic field—or situation—was conceptualized as interactive relatedness, that is, the influence of analyst and patient on each other when in one another's presence (Stern, 2015). Fromm's emphasis on the ways the social and political constitute the foundation for personality and character development complemented Thompson's and Sullivan's views. It also propelled the efforts of those in what came to be called "the interpersonal tradition" to include the sociohistorical influences on the problems of daily living that patients brought to their analysts (Cortina, 2024). By 1948, WAWI had established a clinic to serve individuals with limited incomes (Frie & Sauvayre, 2022).

But psychoanalysis was a field that both welcomed and rejected immigrants depending on when they immigrated to the United States. The first wave embraced institutes as substitute homes and ensconced Freudian principles as havens that offered continuity to their experience. The second wave, more influenced by the Frankfurt School and the emergent social sciences, encountered the first group's orthodoxy as a wall of tradition that called into question their beliefs about the centrality of culture in forging personality (Aiello, 2009). Refused entry to institute training programs and to the American Psychoanalytic Association, those analysts interested in community practice founded their own institutes but were marginalized until resolution of a lawsuit in 1989 that permitted them entry to APsaA. Subsequent renewal of the legacy bequeathed to them by Freud in 1918 and the Free Clinic Movement in Europe has involved a long, arduous journey (Danto, 2005; Harris, 2019).[1]

> Participating in community work essentially requires managing two communities—the external public community ("the world") and the community of psychoanalysts, who constitute the culture of psychoanalytic institutes and associations ("the field").

The Evolution of Community Psychoanalytic Practice

Although critics of psychoanalysis have often assumed the field was suffering from reminiscences, individual psychoanalysts began revising and reformulating both theory and practice to conform to new research on how the mind is situated in a cultural context and within neurobiological constraints (Pivnick, 2013). Analysts interested in how the field's evolving ideas could be applied to projects outside the institute began integrating social, political, and ideological perspectives with intersubjective clinical consultation to systematize the field of community psychoanalysis, emphasizing the role of collaboration in working with community members (González & Peltz, 2021). Hassinger and Pivnick (2022) also highlight the crucial redefinition of the analyst's role to include clinician, consultant, and citizen.

The Significance of Group Relations

In community psychoanalysis as theorized and applied by González and Peltz (2021), "collaboration defines the potential space between two participant organizations: the community health agency and the psychoanalytic institute" (p. 417). Essential to this endeavor is a desire to effect change by supporting and developing community practitioners, both those already working within community organizations and those within the analytic institute. To cultivate an ethos of mutual benefit and learning, projects are conceived as joint initiatives aimed at shared learning and mutual exchange. The collaborative potential space that ensues forms an *operative field*. However, the "field" tends to arise among groups and organizations rather than between individuals. This process stimulates the emergence of a social unconscious, revealed through the complexities of group membership and institutional networks, which, in turn, are influenced by larger sociocultural forces (Hopper, 2003, 2009; Hopper & Weinberg, 2011; Layton, 2020). For the psychoanalytic practitioner group, the community problems and beliefs enter both via *shared activities* and via unconscious *parallel processes*; for the community professionals and participant groups, psychoanalytic ideas and experiences enter through both *explicit training* and via *implicit aspects of group processes*.

Volkan (2013), in his work on large groups, proposed that shared group and community identifications and fantasies establish a "second skin" for individuals, providing them with a feeling of coherence and balance in the world. When groups are disrupted, their wish to find common cause can become even more intense. Consequently, community analysts were instructed to demonstrate, through action, that they can apply psychoanalytic theory to benefit all participants in the groups with whom they are collaborating. "*Showing through action*" defines what is meant by "*operative*" (González & Peltz, 2021; Rudden & Twemlow, 2013; Tubert-Oklander & Hernández de Tubert, 2004).

> The creation of a *procedural "social unconscious"* enhances the mentalizing capacities of communities, helping them develop a capacity for systems intelligence. Consequently, *work on such applied psychoanalytic projects requires establishing clear operational definitions and procedures.*

Operationalizing Collaborative Community Action

When bringing psychoanalytic expertise to projects outside the consulting room (that is, non-clinical settings) and in collaboration with various members of communities and other professionals on projects, practitioners aim to increase capacity of members of highly stressed communities to work on community-based problems, contribute relevant professional expertise, identify and help to obtain needed resources, and to collaborate on planning interventions that can ameliorate ongoing (often intergenerational) effects of natural and human-made disasters, including systemic racism and other forms of dehumanization. Areas of expertise of particular significance might include: intergenerational trauma and impacts on communities; culturally appropriate theories of child development, community and group dynamics/relations; understandings of systemic/structural racism; models of collaboration/consultation; and program/intervention planning and development.

How, though, does one go about an intervention with community groups? This is a particularly thorny question since most psychoanalysts have not studied group dynamics despite the fact that much of our training and professional activities occur in groups (Cushman, 2015; Dalal, 1998; González, 2020; Pivnick & Reading, 2024). In fact, American psychoanalysis has almost entirely neglected *the group*, even as we recognize that psychological development is fostered in the crucible of multiple experiences of membership in groups and surrounding communities. By connecting individuals with *tasks* and *missions* that directly address the needs and problems of the larger society, groups are often underappreciated and undertheorized sites for adult development. While struggling in groups with often chaotic interpersonal impingements, we can develop resilient identities, concern and compassion for others, and a public/political voice (Erikson, 1959, 1963, 1968, 1994a, 1994b; Hassinger & Pivnick, 2022; Tubert-Oklander, 2014).[2]

The Psychoanalytic Community Collaboratory

To address these omissions and challenges for practitioners who work within (or want to work within) community settings, Jane Hassinger and I launched, in 2014, a facilitated web-based seminar, project incubator, and experiential laboratory—the Psychoanalytic Community Collaboratory—which was informed by relational and group psychoanalytic frameworks that highlight group process, multiplicity, intersectionality, historical trauma, enactment, and mourning (Bion, 2003; Bromberg, 1998; Dalal, 1998; Holmes, 2016; Pivnick, 2017a; Salberg & Grand, 2016). Facilitation of the group was guided by democratic-humanistic values and norms that prioritized the value of all members' contributions, differences, and conflicts, as well as empowerment (Berman & Hassinger, 2012; Glassman, 2008; Hassinger & Pivnick, 2021, 2022; Pivnick & Hassinger, 2022). Each Collaboratory session was linked to a curriculum of readings, members' evolving projects, and group process observation.

As the five webinars proceeded, Collaboratory participants created temporary communities in which the value of all voices (Glassman, 2008) as well as their concern for, and mutual implication in, struggles and successes of all were foregrounded (Layton, 2020; Rothberg, 2019). As members increasingly "took up roles" in the group (Shapiro, 2019; Shapiro & Carr, 1991), a sense of "self-in-the group and group-in-the-self" could be felt. Inspired by Eng and Han's (2000) "psychic citizen"—an individual psychic development based on the immigrant's struggle to preserve melancholic identifications during the process of assimilation—we termed this intersubjectively constructed self-state the "*relational citizen*." Within this inherently relational experience, freighted with historical trauma and culturally normative unconscious processes (Layton, 2013, 2020), members revealed increased capacities for multiplicity, empathy, and interpersonal perspective-taking (Davoine & Gaudillière, 2005; Holmes, 2016; Hopper, 2003; Salberg & Grand, 2016; Pivnick & Hassinger, 2022).

The remainder of this paper describes a collaborative community project undertaken by the WAWI's Center for Public Mental Health (CPMH) that applied the Collaboratory practice principles and methodology.

Community Psychoanalysis and Public Mental Health

It is probably not coincidental that many of the community projects undertaken by WAWI have involved work with immigrants and survivors of mass trauma. As early as 1895, Freud understood that many of the symptomatic difficulties patients brought to treatment came from unresolved trauma, which remained unconscious and needed to be connected to conscious memories and words (Ainslie, 2013). Then, in the complex aftermath of the Holocaust, the World Wars of the 20th century, and apartheid, more than the unearthing of individual memory was called for. Indeed, issues of remembrance of collective traumas became a moral imperative (Bohleber, 2007; Gerson, 2009). Publicly bearing witness to testimony through communal memorialization began to be foregrounded in the healing process (O'Loughlin, 2014; Pivnick & Hennes, 2014). The catastrophic collective events we summarized as 9/11, COVID, and the opiate epidemic further reminded us of the need for community intervention since trauma produced predictable distortions to symbolization, group functioning, affective communication, and institutional processes (Pivnick, 2015, 2021). Repairing group polarization, integrating fragmented identities, and reestablishing a sense of agency assumed urgent proportions in both clinical and public imaginaries (Ainslie, 2013; Caruth, 1996; Gobodo-Madikizela, 2015, 2024).

Community-Level Manifestations of Trauma

Traumatized communities, like traumatized individuals, can suffer grievous loss of the ability to comprehend the enormity of what and who was lost. This results, in part, from binary thinking in both their leaders and citizens. After a mass traumatic event like war or foreign incursion—or following multiple generations of unremitting poverty and the family dysfunction it causes—the world tends to be perceived as either good or bad, black or white, but rarely both at once because the ability to hold mixed feelings is one of the capacities that is knocked out by traumatic levels of terror (Pivnick, 2011, 2013, 2015, 2017b). When thinking is reduced to polarities and losses cannot be mourned, a large group, like an individual, is vulnerable to repeating compulsively what is not remembered and represented symbolically (Volkan, 2013). When members of society take in dissociated but enacted trauma, it can also be transmitted transgenerationally (Davoine & Gaudillière, 2005; Salberg & Grand, 2016; Vaughans, 2016).

Post-traumatic fracturing into good-bad polarized thinking also influences how smaller groups function (Hopper, 2003). Specifically, traumatized helplessness induces group incohesion, leaving groups without the capacity to function harmoniously, solve problems, or relate to leaders in a way that results in the completion of tasks or the protection and empowerment of members. The give-and-take even among members of high-functioning groups also diminishes, so solutions are poorly conceived. Perhaps after traumatic events, our unbearable annihilation anxieties stimulate attempts to soothe ourselves through increased boundedness, but the resulting projection of unacceptable feelings also results in our vulnerability being projected, reversed, racialized, and managed with guilt that is denied systematically. Unless powerful subgroups reclaim their projections and acknowledge their own vulnerabilities, polarization intensifies, manifesting in the scapegoating of socially vulnerable groups (Davids, 2002, 2011).

Over time, and more recently, the many deaths from 9/11, COVID, and opioids hit polarized communities. The ensuing processes, especially when fanned by politicians, clarify how binaries can settle into a pattern of grievance versus grief.[3] This is not a bug but a feature of trauma and recovery after a mass traumatic event. At such times, we need leaders to provide flexible containment that permits cycling between dismantling established forms and creating absence; and constructing new forms as a presence—reminding ourselves that all structures both appear and disappear and will inevitably cycle back to something that needs further transformation (Hagman, 2015; Pivnick, 2017a).[4]

The Importance of Dialogue and Relational Healing

The first step in repairing the capacity for thinking, communicating, and taking up citizenship roles after communal or intergenerational trauma involves dialogue with another person or another subjectivity (Beebe et al., 2013; Boulanger, 2011; Davoine & Gaudillière, 2005;

Pivnick, 2011, 2013; Pivnick & Hennes, 2014). We learn others' emotional meanings through being exposed to their stories, which in turn helps us to predict behavior, diminish anxiety and paranoia, and build trust (Stern, 2010). Whereas in psychotherapy, this dialogue arises with the therapist, in community psychoanalysis, conversation occurs among subgroups.

By 2022, of the many groups who were pushed out of the mainstream imaginary through a process of group splitting, the asylum-seeking families and children with disabilities needing services for learning in public schools drew increasing attention from the politicians and media. An article in the *New York Times Magazine* (Closson, 2023) about one community institution that tried to address these massive needs came to the attention of the WAWI CPMH. In a Brooklyn pilot begun in 2017, P.S. 15 began to serve students with intellectual disabilities, who had difficulty finding the services they needed in public schools and instead left for specialized private schools. Two teachers typically led a class, which usually included a small group of general education students and approximately four children following special education plans, along with one paraprofessional per child. Unlike many other programs for students with disabilities, this program was inclusive. When CPMH's research revealed the school also included some of the surging asylum-seeking students, we speculated they might benefit from our assistance with managing these two groups of students, who had likely experienced much trauma, neglect, and alienation, and that P.S. 15 would be a welcoming place for relational ideas about learning, classroom dynamics, and co-creation of a program to address these. We came to call the emerging program the Schools as Refuge Project.

The Schools as Refuge Project: Genesis and Context

On a blustery fall day in 2023, holding a takeout coffee in hand, I entered the bright red double doors of P.S. 15, a preschool to fifth-grade school in Red Hook, Brooklyn. I was accompanied on that day by Dr. Beryl Nightingale, a clinical psychologist, child analyst, and neuropsychologist, whom I had worked with for many years at the WAWI. We represented the newly reconstituted CPMH, which had a history of working on training mental health evaluators and attorneys on expert witness procedures and had published a manual, now in its second edition due to its popularity, for the Appleseed Network on working with asylum-seekers (Nardone & Casado-Frankel, 2025). Headed initially by Dr. Kimberlyn Leary and more recently chaired by Dr. Maria Nardone, the Center was now to be chaired by me and advised by one of our WAWI trustees, Mr. Tom Hennes. We recognized that our mission was to respond to emerging sociopolitical issues that create distress and trauma in communities by working with communities' existing resources and partnerships, applying our relational and interpersonal knowledge and practices to enhance public mental health.

Building the Collaborative Team

After much discussion and in consultation with the Institute's Board of Trustees, chaired by Dr. Mary McRae, led by Dr. Elizabeth Krimendahl, and the Social Impact Committee headed by Dr. Jack Drescher, we had decided to create a program that would build on the former work with asylum-seeking families, but add a new twist. Educators who encountered these often-traumatized students in their classrooms needed support and training. *Studies suggested that socio-emotional approaches to learning would help reduce intensified anxiety, loneliness, and uncertainty* (Abramson, 2022; Brackett & Cipriano, 2020; Pothireddy, 2024). This was something we were well-equipped to provide.

However, studies have also shown that traditional Social-Emotional Learning (SEL) approaches might not suffice for students entrenched in adversity, necessitating a more nuanced and culturally sensitive framework to meet their emotional needs effectively. Despite available professional development, many programs remained disconnected from the lived realities of Black and Latino students, leaving their needs unmet. These students, though resilient, often faced challenges that conventional SEL strategies fail to address. For example, a child raised in an environment filled with violence and neglect may find it difficult to relate to SEL activities that presume stable family structures, access to emotional support, and high verbal functioning. This disconnect highlighted the urgent need for SEL initiatives to be modified to become more culturally responsive and adaptable to the diverse realities of our students (Elbakoury, 2024; Forner, 2018; Jose, 2024).

Building an Alliance

Entering the school system as great experts, saviors, or heroes would be ill-advised. Did the school even want our "help"? The educators were far more knowledgeable about the needs and problems in their neighborhood and at their school than we were. Developing a project to reduce anxiety and the behavioral disruptiveness that it can create in classrooms, we would require a team with varied expertise. My experience in educational settings, program development, and community psychoanalysis would be useful. I had founded a school in the 1970s, consulted for schools, and published several papers on how psychoanalysis could be applied in a school setting. I had also co-created with Dr. Jane Hassinger the Psychoanalytic Community Collaboratory to support mental health professionals working in diverse community settings. Other members of the Schools as Refuge Project team were similarly experienced in practicing in this sort of setting. Nightingale's private practice, the Heights Psychology Collective, had brought her into contact with many schools and educational professionals. As a Department of Education (DOE) vendor, she was in a unique position to develop this pilot program with me and, in fact, worked with someone who recommended the principal of P.S. 15 as someone who had devoted her school resources to providing special education placements for even severely disabled students and for the large number of asylum-seeking children being bused to New York City from Texas.

Let me introduce you to the other players on our CPMH Schools as Refuge Project team, all experienced with work in diverse community settings: Dr. Sheri-Ann Cowie, a psychologist on the faculty of Yale University and the Group Relations Institute, who already had an expertise in working with schools from an organizational perspective, proved to be instrumental in organizing our group relations analysis. Dr. Brooke Marlin, a candidate in the Child Adolescent Psychotherapy Training Program, who was bilingual and worked with families and asylum-seekers in Queens, brought to our attention the book *The Rabbit Listened* by Cori Doerrfeld (2018), which became a key organizing motif. Dr. Victoria Malkin, a faculty member at WAWI, joined us in the second year. As a parent in the neighborhood whose children had attended the school, she had also done work with the criminal justice system in Red Hook and knew the school well. Crucially, Dr. Howard

Steele, head of the Center for Attachment Research at The New School and, by coincidence, an analytic candidate at WAWI, agreed to help us with the data-gathering and management portion of the project.[5] On the P.S. 15 team, in addition to Principal Julie Cavanagh, were the community liaison coordinator, Ms. Deresie Pierre, the school social workers, Ms. Gillian Chimera Stass and Ms. Dalila Mendez, and several guidance counselors, as well as the District Head of Social Work, Ms. Valeria Ossa.

Understanding the Community Context: Red Hook, Brooklyn

Red Hook, Brooklyn, is a neighborhood with a complex blend of multigenerational poverty, public housing, industrial history, and rapid gentrification. Recent traumas—including the murder of the school's former principal, ongoing recovery from Superstorm Sandy, and the aftereffects of the COVID-19 pandemic—created additional (often unconscious) layers of stress for both students and educators. During initial site visits, it also became clear that paraprofessional aides ("paras") were essential to classroom functioning. This discovery prompted a revision of the project's focus. Instead of targeting children directly, the CPMH team would support teachers and paraprofessionals in managing classroom dynamics and promoting emotional regulation by creating listening partnerships among the individuals and groups.

The Eight Stages of Co-creation: A Framework for Collaborative Intervention

We structured our intervention using an eight-stage model for inclusive community program development. This approach was informed by publicly available resources from Switchboard (2024), a refugee resettlement agency, alongside our own experience within the Psychoanalytic Community Collaboratory and the Psychoanalytic Institute of Northern California's perspective on community psychoanalysis. The latter emphasizes the importance of analyzing both the target community and the psychoanalytic community of consultants (González & Peltz, 2021).

Co-creation places clients at the heart of the design process, supporting the development of innovative products and inclusive programs without a single "owner." The benefits include deeper insights into the needs of specific populations, increased success in addressing community needs from the outset, and more effective integration of content and technology. The process begins with empathic listening, which generates insights that help providers develop and select ideas to prototype. Providers and community members then refine these ideas through an *iterative* process—revising and re-prototyping until a workable prototype is ready for community feedback. This cycle continues through ongoing consultation until a viable final product is achieved.

Stage 1: Listening Sessions

Our consultations began with listening to key community members, such as CPMH practitioners, P.S. 15 administrators, district social work leaders, teachers, and our research partners at The New School's Center for Attachment Research. This stage emphasized building alliances and deeply understanding the community's lived experience. We identified several key issues: developmental delays resulting from COVID-19, trauma affecting asylum-seeking and refugee students, and the need for safe, supportive environments. We approached our work with curiosity, humility, and empathy.

During our initial in-person meeting, we learned about the school's concerns regarding students affected by COVID-related development delays and the long-standing impact of multigenerational poverty on educational attainment. As discussed above, these issues were more significant than anticipated. Asylum-seeking families were frequently relocated due to changing city protocols, resulting in lengthy commutes and unexplained absences. These students faced the challenge of learning English while managing trauma responses disruptive to their learning and that of their peers. Our assessment revealed that both groups—asylum-seekers and students with disabilities—required a sense of safety and containment within the school.

We also considered the neighborhood's unique context: once home to dockworkers, its small enclaves were shaped by ethnic and socioeconomic differences. The area included housing projects, a harbor beach, public amenities, and a mix of long-term low-income residents and newer, wealthier families attracted by proximity to Manhattan. Several team members had personal experience with the community, which further informed our understanding and fueled our curiosity about the school's needs and our potential contributions as relative outsiders.

First impressions in community work, as in clinical work, are significant. The school's familiar environment—with student artwork and public-school hallmarks like large clocks—contrasted with heightened security protocols due to recent violence and ongoing trauma from the pandemic and the murder of the principal. The community was also still recovering from Superstorm Sandy, with ongoing disruptions a decade later.

A school tour provided key insights: every classroom had both engaged students and multiple paraprofessional teachers ("paras") assigned to children with disabilities, making up about half the teaching staff. We questioned their training, support, and collaboration with teachers. Learning that paras were only paired with children with disabilities (not asylum-seeking children) led us to shift focus from students to supporting teachers and paraprofessionals. As highlighted by Dobrich in this volume, revising one's hypotheses resembles the move from unformulated to formulated experience in psychoanalytic work.

Deeper understanding of the students—especially asylum-seekers and children with disabilities —revealed that many faced trauma, displacement, and language barriers, impacting their emotional self-regulation and overall well-being (Wyatt & Beznes, 2026). Most of the students with disabilities were on the autism spectrum, nonverbal, and highly sensitive to classroom disruptions.

We also sought to understand better teachers and paraprofessional aides, who were largely underpaid people of color (Will, 2022). Administrators noted they lacked adequate training and support for managing classroom emotional crises. It became clear that providing teachers and paraprofessionals with effective social and emotional strategies was crucial for supporting children while managing the needs of other students, many from families with their own traumatic histories. We concluded that the school community was not so much overwhelmed by conflict as starved for resources. This finding guided our next steps: learning more about the resources the community needed and could use, and determining which needs we could address.

Stage 2: Contextual Needs Assessment

We conducted a comprehensive assessment to identify a "good problem" within the community—an issue that warranted a fresh perspective and could benefit from collaborative intervention. This involved creating questions and framing issues at a broad level, allowing the deeper needs and desires of the community to emerge. Importantly, *this stage was conducted* ***with*** *the community, not just* ***for*** *them.*

To measure our effectiveness, we selected reliable pre- and post-intervention tools, choosing the teacher self-efficacy instrument described by Skaalvik and Skaalvik (2010). The principal highlighted the value of attachment theory-based supervision for training counselors and teachers, emphasizing the importance of understanding personal attachment histories to foster openness and alternative approaches, which led us to search for a measure of reflective functioning (mentalization). We identified two key student groups: those from asylum-seeking families and those experiencing multigenerational poverty and trauma. While multiple agencies supported migrant children (New York City Department of Education, 2022), faculty and staff needs were largely unaddressed. Limited volunteer resources meant that individual therapy or class consultations were not feasible.[6] Therefore, our intervention aimed to improve student learning and well-being by enhancing the emotional regulation and self-efficacy of teachers, paraprofessionals, and administrators.

Stage 3: Formulating Insights

Our central insight, shared with CPMH and the school team, was that *supporting teachers' and school staff's ability to identify and manage trauma responses in themselves and their students would help traumatized children learn and succeed.* Research showed that increased emotional regulation, driven by improved teacher/aide self-efficacy, led to higher student cognitive achievement (Fonagy, 1991; Fonagy et al., 2017, 2018; Pivnick & Hassinger, 2021; Thapa et al., 2013). Untrained adults were vulnerable to being triggered by students' stress reactions, resulting in decreased effectiveness and increased burnout. Thus, our goal became providing interpersonal-relational training to help staff co-regulate emotions and stress, fostering greater efficacy, job satisfaction, and retention (Dietrich, 2021). Based on the school team's requests, we proposed a series of six initial workshops for teachers and paras.

Stage 4: Connecting the Community to Resources and Tools

In this stage, we partnered with the community to establish a core co-creation group and identify resources. Collaborative decision-making was emphasized to empower the community to take ownership of the project. We developed and tailored training materials on attachment theory, trauma, and affect regulation for the school context. Recommended readings included an attachment-based framework for learning difficulties and teaching strategies (Boldt & Pivnick, 2013).

We engaged with other school principals, mental health professionals, and educational psychologists, including Dr. Jonathan Cohen of the School Climate Research Center and Columbia University Teachers College. Regular meetings with Drs. Howard and Miriam Steele from the Center for Attachment Research at The New School assisted us in determining the most valuable theoretical and practical components for this setting.

Key principles to be communicated to teachers and paras included the importance of caregivers' capacity to manage their own and others' emotions and the concept of the reflective functioning that underpins the transmission of child attachment (Menashe-Grinberg et al., 2022; Steele & Steele, 2018). Training sessions, based on their research, were designed to model reflectiveness and mentalization, using real-life situations to elicit authentic feelings and promote reflective functioning. We also adapted materials on immigration stress that included free online resources and webinars about managing trauma in refugee children (Switchboard, 2023).

Stage 5: Developing Collaborative Prototypes

Community-based models were developed to illustrate how the final product would look and function. Continuous feedback loops among contributors helped refine designs and concepts. Our group reviewed an adapted video presentation originally created by the Steeles' lab students for "Clowns without Borders", an NGO serving refugees internationally, modifying it to be trauma- and attachment-sensitive for our context.[7] We incorporated case studies relevant to children with learning challenges and autism spectrum disorder and included principles from Polyvagal Theory (Daniels, 2023; Porges, 2011) for affect regulation in classrooms.

A three-workshop framework emerged: the first introduced all participants; the second facilitated discussion of practice principles; and the third applied these ideas to real classroom dilemmas. Issues addressed included parent engagement, disruptive behaviors, conflicts among students, gentrification-related stresses, entitlement, and self-doubt. Participants developed both inner and interpersonal listening skills, paralleling their goals as educators and reflecting the principles of individual psychotherapy.

Stage 6: Public User Testing

At this stage, the product was refined based on public user feedback to determine whether the "good problem" was being addressed. Workshop feedback highlighted areas for improvement, such as increasing diverse representation in visual materials and incorporating pauses and discussions to enhance engagement and relevance. The team adjusted content pacing and developed breakout activities to facilitate meaningful contributions.

Stage 7: Implementation

The nearly finished product was introduced to the broader community for further feedback. We identified the physical space, facilitators, time frames, and volunteers for the implementation. The Schools as Refuge Project team, together with Howard Steele and graduate student volunteers, led Zoom workshops, some of which were attended by the school's guidance staff. Workshop timing and breakout room prompts were organized in advance.

Stage 8: Assessment and Reflection

We established a formalized process to assess workshop viability and gather data on how well the intervention addressed community needs. We considered how the co-creation process and its outcomes might inform future research and development. The Skaalvik and Skaalvik (2010) *Teacher Self-Efficacy Scale* was administered by New School graduate students and analyzed in Qualtrics. Participant feedback questionnaires were also used to evaluate progress and inform future initiatives. The Skaalviks scale assessed teacher burnout and self-efficacy within the broader school context and individually. Pre-workshop evaluations indicated strong belief in the school's ability to create a safe, inclusive atmosphere even in challenging classes. The *Perceived School Context Subscale* highlighted high levels of supervisory support, positive parent relations, and teacher autonomy. We also kept process notes to analyze community group dynamics, and subgroup trends were tracked. As initially sensed, the school community already possessed significant strengths.

The First Year Project: Tailoring Interventions for Faculty Groups

From initial (pilot) workshops that were held in May and June of 2024 to identify needs, measure baselines on reliable and valid scales of teacher self-efficacy, and increase understanding of emotional regulation in teachers/aides, we gathered data and created an alliance that allowed us to begin a regular schedule of groups for teachers, professional aides, and related service providers in fall 2024 that continued for two years.

We learned from our early data that the paras and teachers had slightly different learning styles and preferences, with the teachers more responsive to content and the paras preferring discussion-based information. We used this conclusion both to guide our curriculum planning, workshop design, and for considerations of group relations that impact on listening partnerships.

With our school partners, we decided that the focus for the second year would be on professional identity building and mutual support. In a vote of confidence, the school secured DOE funding to pay the paras for additional workshops.

The Second Year Project

The second-year, six-workshop curriculum was delivered experientially to a group of 15 paras. To foster trust and listening, we aimed to build alliances among the participants, who had never worked together and were unfamiliar with one another, despite each working with similar students in separate classrooms.

During the workshops, which built on one another, we introduced stress management techniques, as well as self and mutual regulation strategies. We also created a curriculum to develop a deeper awareness of how their personal attachment histories influenced how they responded to their students' struggles, and of how autism spectrum disorder influenced their students' reactions and could, in turn, be affected by their attuned responses. We taught the use of adapted breathing and group movement exercises to regulate arousal in a classroom, as well as how to identify and label emotions in their own and their students' behavior.[8] We structured dyadic listening and nonverbal mirroring exercises and helped them re-define their job responsibilities as professional skills.

Throughout the workshops, we emphasized the importance of play. For instance, we used bubble blowing to teach breathing techniques, a stretch exercise band held by the entire group while mirroring one another's movements to model elasticity and spontaneity, and a (dry) drinking game of "Adverbs" assisted them in learning verbal labels for emotions and behaviors. The latter exercise was a fun way to address their understandable discouragement: managing nonverbal students in predominantly verbal classrooms was extremely challenging. Over time, participation and enthusiasm increased, but for much of the year, the groups exhibited resistance through what Bion (2003) would call a "fight-flight" dynamic, frequently coming late, leaving early, or choosing not to participate verbally.

The Second Year: Empowerment and Professionalization

A significant outcome of this process was both an improved ability to work reflectively and implicitly, and, as they watched one another grow and change, they felt our support for their emotional connection to their students. As time went on, they developed more self-awareness and spoke respectfully of each other's work. Fewer people arrived late; by the end, they worked together and with us to craft an actual job description that reflected their role in professionally managing their students' emotional regulation—something they had never been given before, even at hiring. We then took on the role of advocates (modeling a sense of agency) by delivering the job description to the school administration. Despite continuing reluctance to publicly expose their personal data, a few did record and share with us five-minute reflections on how their work had changed during our joint project.[9]

Although the paras' reflective functioning scores showed room for improvement, some clearly were using emotion regulation tools from our workshops. We also noticed their deployment of affectionate but charged humor in a new way: the principal began announcing our arrival by calling us the "fancy therapists from the city." She, too, had joined the fight, but in a way that acknowledged our role as valued outsiders and the paras' valued "insider" professional responsibilities—for which she was paying them to become more expert. Best of all, the conflict was being expressed in words as well as action.

Group Relations Findings and Challenges

Reflections on the workshops overall yielded a number of insights. I will group these into three themes, Authority/Crisis; Interpersonal/Intergroup Dynamics, and Parallel Processes. First, I will detail issues related to authority, which is typically the first issue to arise in groups. The school was highly organized but also in constant crisis. Sometimes scheduled meetings would have to be canceled due to emergencies; in one Zoom workshop, the principal suddenly "disappeared" to take an emergency phone call, but did so without notifying the group, which delayed the start of the meeting; one afternoon she had to stay after school for many hours with a child in crisis because there was no other Crisis Team staff available and the ACS worker was delayed in picking up the child. It felt to us as if it were a firehouse in which the administration was in the role of firefighters, putting out fires. The principal was extraordinarily skilled and available to distressed teachers and students, but in working that way, she also introduced inconsistency to teamwork.

Next, I will share some observations about interpersonal and intergroup relations. We noticed divisions between the teachers as a group and the paraprofessionals as a group, with the teachers feeling more identified with the principal, while the paraprofessionals showed ambivalence about their roles and sometimes defied rules, such as those related to promptness.

For a workshop addressing refugee trauma reactions, we developed a curriculum related to the expectation that students might experience high anxiety and dislocation: we provided them with reassuring phrases in several languages. However, the teachers told us their anxiety was triggered more by students' unexpected absences, experienced as disappearances, than by outbursts or disruptive behaviors.

When discussing their hyperarousal, we were shocked to hear that many teachers and paras were still experiencing PTSD symptoms from the Superstorm Sandy floods that devastated the neighborhood five years earlier, which were only now being addressed by the city. We correctly anticipated post-COVID developmental delays but were less prepared for signs of ambiguous loss caused by sudden displacements due to rising rents, grocery prices, and gentrification of their impoverished neighborhood.[10] Recent arrivals through gentrification tended to be wealthier students placed in the dual-language program; the paras for the lower-functioning students were envious of those who served in those classes. Less frustrated and disruptive, these students were observed by administrators to behave instead with entitlement (e.g., impatience to be at the front of the line; refusal to play with long-standing neighborhood kids; occasional flight-or-fight reactions while adjusting to a new neighborhood where they felt they did not belong) but were more accessible through words.

Reflecting on our own parallel process, we realized that the CPMH was also experiencing splits. The most noticeable was the division between the board, which had not yet succeeded in initiating fundraising, and the CPMH itself. A second, still troubling split existed within the CPMH between frontline consultants and our essential support partners, who acted as a third but sometimes appeared less engaged.[11] It was clear that we were enacting some form of parallel process with the school, a fact highlighted by my own feelings of being overwhelmed and under-resourced, which were in line with those of the principal.

Sustaining and Expanding the Initiative

To aid in the implementation of new learning, we decided together with the school leadership team to continue to provide support for the school leaders in the form of observations and to attend to unconscious parallel processes in their team and ours. If funding were secured for a third year of operation, we hope to focus on building teacher-para partnerships. Although we expected to encounter *capacity* and *boundary* issues emphasizing the importance of ***containment***, and to be able to provide holding for them during unexpected (crises) events, what we discovered during implementation was that we, too, were at capacity. Fewer candidates were available to volunteer than I expected. The principal and I felt similarly deluged.

Continuing Challenges: Institutional Contexts

Despite many successful outcomes, challenges remained as we tried integrating the project within established institutional structures. Volunteer fatigue, lack of visibility, and insufficient fundraising were ongoing hurdles at WAWI, paralleling the struggles faced by the school community in securing resources and recognition. Furthermore, this appeared to be a parallel process to the dynamics in the P.S. 15 community, who all reported feeling "gaslit" and continually let down by the government agencies that were meant to support them. At WAWI, we noted an institutional social structure that led to a parallel split between the actual consultants and those who took on more supervisory functions. During our end-of-school-year visit with the school team, we shared our observations of their team and ours and began a discussion about how to address those issues. One issue identified more clearly at this stage led to an animated discussion about how to handle wealth disparities, particularly the effect of entitled students and families on the school culture while maintaining fairness.

> We reluctantly concluded that an institute may not be the best place to generate social action, because candidates rotate through quickly and are generally quite strapped for time beyond their educational goals.

The CPMH decided to broaden our mission to include project incubation and the study of community psychoanalysis; in this way, we would not require additional project development or fundraising, but could expand participation and engagement beyond volunteer activists. While renewing our commitment to making a social impact and to collaborative practice, we hoped to build awareness in the WAWI community of the many ways available to reach beyond narrowly defined boundaries. One additional project we fostered was a book by Dr. Ken Barish (2024) on coping with political polarization called *Bridging Our Political Divide: How Liberals and Conservatives Can Understand Each Other and Find Common Ground.*

In a welcome development, by the end of our second year of operations at the school, the WAWI Board of Trustees hired a group of consultants of their own to plan a program to increase public visibility for the institute and its programs with an eye to future fundraising efforts. The *Schools as Refuge Project* was featured in its presentation deck as one of the two most compelling and mission-aligned programs. The report highlighted its social impact and commended CPMH's commitment to upholding WAWI's legacy and values. Furthermore, in another sign of our growing perceived legitimacy, we were invited to present our work at the institute's clinical case conference. It was clear that both the school and institute communities had undergone some degree of transformation during this community psychoanalytic collaboration. As of this writing, we await the results of fundraising efforts.

Reflections on the Co-Creation Process

The project demonstrated the value of psychoanalytic listening and group work in addressing contemporary educational and social challenges. By fostering reflective partnerships and mutual support, the initiative contributed to the growth of "relational citizens" and strengthened democratic group functioning. Close collaboration led to a high level of engagement on CPMH and at P.S. 15, keener empathic insight into the community's needs, and success in accommodating those needs from the outset. However, despite its beneficial collective results, it also proved to be a slow and humbling process, particularly because it relied heavily on volunteer efforts.

However, as in any interpersonal, intersubjective project, the resources that had to be recruited were also internal.

> The reflective aspect of the process, particularly gaining perspective through writing, was a key component of the operational field and should be considered a stage of operationalization.

As I was reminded and have learned on past projects, it is at this stage that splits are often enacted within or between writers (or writers and editors). It is important to resolve them by formulating their meanings in paradoxical rather than binary form (Pivnick, 2017b). As in individual psychoanalysis, connecting the disconnected emotions and thoughts in an updated, more dialectical formulation is crucial to the consultation process.

As I was finishing my final text, I noticed I was slowed by my disappointment that the Schools as Refuge Project had been unable to complete the project as envisioned. My writing kept reverting to overly idealized descriptions despite my knowledge of the fundamental constraints on our work. Once I acknowledged my grief to the editor, I could better formulate the narrative arc in less triumphal form.

One missed stitch continued to bother me. I did not have an adequate way to understand all the enacted group dynamics in our workshops. How did the principal's enacted disappearance from her role in the workshop, the teachers' distress about the children's disappearances, and the enacted erasure of the paras' competence and job description relate to one another? An internet search for historical news of the murdered principal provided a new way to formulate an answer to that puzzle. What felt during the workshops as if it had happened just before Superstorm Sandy in 2012 actually happened 33 years earlier, in 1992! At the time, a distraught nine-year-old kid had disappeared from school, and, in an extraordinary act of devotion, the former principal left the school to try to track down and rescue the student, who lived in the nearby projects. While there, the principal was shot in the crossfire of a gang war.

I believe these "disappearances" were how the event resurfaced in enacted form in the workshops, in part, because the not fully symbolized trauma still reverberated in the community, much as Volkan (2013) has depicted. The group, as "second skin," had been ruptured. As Davids' (2002, 2011) work on internal racism shows, people of color are disproportionately affected after mass traumas due to groups' use of projection to manage feelings of vulnerability. Perhaps this was why the paras were so frequently deemed in need of repair.

The principal's seeming hyper-responsivity to emergencies and the neighborhood population's ongoing intergenerational trauma-inducing role-responsive helplessness and chronic hyperarousal in the school staff also now made sense—in its proper context—as understandable, but perhaps temporally displaced, responses to a past traumatically overstimulating event. It was extreme devotion that propelled the former principal into the peril that led to his death. The history could now be rendered as a cautionary tale rather than a ghost story.

There was yet another wrinkle to account for. In 1992, the neighborhood was terrifyingly violent. Huge investments were made to make the neighborhood more prosperous, in hopes of making it a safer place. IKEA, Fairway, and Amazon moved in to bring jobs. The unanticipated consequence, though, was that the neighborhood's improvements attracted more gentrification, which displaced residents and thereby created new losses—felt even more acutely by those like the paras who were not paid a living wage.

It is an ironic story, but one that is happening all over the world. As we have seen over and over, such dramatically improved prosperity can be destructive to community life. This is an illustration of the repeating cycle of entropy and new growth I referenced earlier in this chapter. The work of community psychoanalysis is never fully completed; rather, it allows the process of transformation to continue in a less impeded fashion.

Conclusion: Moving Together Toward an Uncertain Future

Humans are intrinsically relational—both born into and maturing in group settings. An interpersonal/relational psychoanalytic framework recognizes the psychic and social importance of strengthening our relatedness and enhancing our ability to build and sustain well-functioning, well-led groups in all the settings in which we live and work. As we engage in play and struggle together in communities, we bear witness to our shared histories, mutual concerns, and emotional needs while also growing citizens (Pivnick & Hassinger, 2026; Khetan, 2025; Pivnick & Hassinger, 2022; Stern, 2023).

The pilot project described in this paper was a collaborative effort to help educators cope with post-pandemic pressures stemming from an influx of asylum-seeking students and the pandemic's effects on educators' ability to address intergenerational poverty and learning challenges. It was premised on the idea that developing listening partnerships among all the stakeholders in a school community and between the school community and the psychoanalytic consultants who organized and implemented this intervention would provide beneficial support for their educational mission. As a new network of relationships formed, bringing the school, the institute, and the community closer together, the two groups felt each other's struggles in a way that provided new insights for addressing many shared problems. Exploring whether divisions ensuing from traumatic grief indicated a need for mourning together community losses guided us to a new direction for our work.

Remarkably, this project that transpired over only two years produced notable effects for both the psychoanalytic "field" and the broader "community." Throughout this collaboration, both communities evolved. The school received essential training in trauma-informed and attachment-based teaching. The psychoanalysts gained vital support for a core principle of psychoanalysis that had been difficult to implement due to sociopolitical pressures from the wider world and their own professional ranks. It has been an exciting exercise to reimagine analysts using their listening skills in service of becoming a resource for the community—a fellow citizen and an activist partner in participatory relational citizenship.

Notes

1 Psychoanalytic history is replete with schismatic dynamics. Additional exploration of the reasons for the exclusion of non-physician clinicians and group practitioners can be found in Cushman (1996, 2015) and Makari (2008).

2 Jane Hassinger and I have written several articles and chapters about community psychoanalysis. One, "The Community Turn: Relational Citizenship in the Psychoanalytic Community Collaboratory" (2022), was published in the *International Journal of Psychoanalysis*. Another, "The Relational Citizen as Implicated Subject: Emergent Unconscious Processes in the Psychoanalytic Community Collaboratory" (2023), was published in *Inhabiting Implication in Racial Oppression and Relational Psychoanalysis* (Kabasakalian-McKay & Mark, 2023). Still another, "The Child in the School, the School in the Community, and the Community in the Child: Linking Psychic and Social Domains in School Violence Prevention" (2021), was published in the *International Journal of Applied Psychoanalytic Studies*. A fourth paper, "The 21st Century Psychoanalyst: Clinician, Community Member, and Relational Citizen", was co-presented as an invited talk for the William Alanson White Institute Colloquium on 02/09/24. Finally, our article, "The Work and Play of Democracy: Growing Relational Citizens," was published in March, 2026, in the *International Journal of Applied Psychoanalysis*.

3 I have written in detail about that historical development in a paper on the 20th anniversary of 9/11 published in a 2021 issue of *Psychoanalytic Perspectives*, called "Recollecting the Vanishing Forms of 9/11: Twenty Years of Ruptures, Ripples, and Reflections." I argued the attacks of 9/11 produced the physical collapse of the buildings; the collapse of iconic symbols of our financial power; temporal collapse, as evidenced by the confusion of the meanings of current circumstances with those of the past;

narrative collapse, as shown by our subsequent inability to tell a common story; and intersubjective collapse, as seen in the difficulty we have in trusting others with different viewpoints than our own lest we lose our own valued selfhood.

4 Leaders also need to be mindful that in incohesive groups (Hopper, 2003), with polarized, fragmented, fused, aggregated, or massified subgroups, one faction may be moving from grievance to hope, but other subgroups will be falling from hope into grievance or grief. Thus, healing grievance or grief does not inevitably lead to hope. Although we can transform grievance into grief, hope is a potential byproduct of that process, not an outcome.

5 Additional members of CPMH were Dr. Ken Barish, Dr. Maria Nardone, Dr. Lori Bohm, Dr. Lisa Dubinsky, Dr. Jonathan Cohen, Ms. Lucy Bruell, and Ms. Dan Liu.

6 Another model we considered was Reflective Network Therapy, developed by Dr. Gilbert Kliman (2018) to provide individual mentalization-based therapy to students within a classroom while creating a network of family and community members to support the children and one another. Despite its proven track record, its structure demanded more staffing resources than we had available.

7 Graduate student members of the Steeles' New School Lab, including Ms. Eleana Antonaki and Ms. Robyn Attarian, authored and helped revise the video.

8 We built on the research of Blau and Siegel (1978) on the use of "breathing together" as an adaptive reflex in working with children on the autism spectrum, the research of Cohen (2007, 2014) on mental health clinicians and educators working together, and of Bragin and Bragin (2010) and Cohen et al. (2015) on helping survivors of violence learn through mentalizing emotional meanings in the classroom. An emphasis on improving reflective functioning (Steele & Steele, 2018) also informed our design.

9 This is one example, scored for reflective functioning:

Q1: Tell me about the time your work felt like it was really going well, when you felt really connected to the child. Tell me what happened. happened in that moment.

A: I, being very simple. I, like, stubbed my toe. No, a child ran over my toe. And for the first time, he automatically apologized, normally a kid that didn't really apologize, apologized, like right away, without someone saying, Okay, we need to say sorry now. We just had an accident. It was nice to see that progress and seeing, you know, a hope for a child, that learning that ever since the accident, the right thing that he goes to say is like, sorry. And that, and that was, that was nice. [RF = 4.5 for the reference to a valued normative response from the child when the child spontaneously apologized for running over the adult's toe—reflecting an understanding of the nature of mental states, especially the notion that certain mental states (apologies) are tied to readily acknowledging behaviors (like accidentally hurting another.)]

Q2: Okay. Tell me about a time when you saw the child confused or frustrated, angry or sad, and what was going on.

A: Oh, we were doing work. It was typical, showing his frustration for learning—Oh, I can't do it. I want my mom. And [he was] just having a tantrum. And I decided, well, let me go mirror what a child is doing and see how he reacts. And so I started doing it—like, well, I don't want to do this, and I want my mommy. And he got really quiet and he understood that like, you know, we don't have to act like that. It's okay to have feelings, but we can, you know, translate it in a different and better way. And, you know, he's improved things. [Scoring the speaker for reflective functioning seems to show an understanding of factors that determine affect regulation, and the functionality of RF insofar as it helps one understand why another may be upset, as well as through showing understanding the upset may become regulated. RF = 4 for the partial evidence of this, as the adult's imitation potentially could be felt by the child as "mocking," despite the fact it was intended to show that frustration can be dealt with by the child and the para together (without recourse to seeking out the mother's help). This is one of the developmental considerations of RF and one of the results of our project's focus on listening partnerships.]

10 Ambiguous loss is characterized by a deep sense of loss and sadness similar to those following a death, but not connected to an actual death. It is often accompanied by chronic confusion, uncertainty, and lack of closure (Boss, 2022). Resilience is conferred through finding recognition and making meaning, rather than achieving closure solely through grieving.

11 The "analytic third" is a psychoanalytic term first coined by Thomas Ogden (1994) and elaborated by other relational analysts like Jessica Benjamin (2017)). The term refers to a co-created space between the analyst and patient. The analytic process unfolds in this intersubjective field so that both the patient and analyst are continually shaping it while it is shaping them and change takes place *between* two subjectivities. In this transitional space where meaning is co-created, polarized emotions and ideas can be held in tension, fostering dialectical thinking.

References

Abramson, A. (2022). Children's mental health is in crisis: As pandemic stressors continue, kids' mental health needs to be addressed in schools. *Monitor on Psychology*, *53*(1), 69. https://www.apa.org/monitor/2022/01/special-childrens-mental-health

Aiello, T. (2009). Psychoanalysts in exile. *Psychoanalytic Perspectives*, *6*(2), 8–34. https://doi.org/10.1080/1551806X.2009.10473052

Ainslie, R. (2013). Intervention strategies for addressing collective trauma: Healing communities ravaged by racial strife. *Psychoanalysis, Culture & Society, 18*, 140–152. https://doi.org/10.1057/pcs.2013.3

Altman, N. (2011). *The analyst in the inner city: Race, class, and culture through a psychoanalytic lens*. Routledge.

Barish, K. (2024). *Bridging our political divide: How liberals and conservatives can understand each other and find common ground.* Routledge.

Beebe, B., McCrorie, E., & Pivnick, B. (December, 2013). Poetry of 9/11: Trauma, grief, and imagination. *Clio's Psyche: Understanding the "Why" of Culture, Current Events, History, and Society. (Special Issue on Poetry and Psychohistory), 20*(3), 314–323.

Benjamin, J. (2017). *Beyond doer and done to: Recognition theory, intersubjectivity and the third.* Routledge.

Berman, K. S., & Hassinger, J. A. (2012). Women on purpose: Interrogating a model for cross-cultural, interdisciplinary collaborations. In Georgina Tsolidis (Eds.), *Identities in transition* (pp. 167–179). Brill. https://doi.org/10.1163/9781848880825_017

Bermudez, G. (2019). Community psychoanalysis: A contribution to an emerging paradigm. *Psychoanalytic Inquiry, 39*(5), 297–304. ihttps://doi.org/10.1080/07351690.2019.1623582

Bion, W. R. (2003). *Experiences in groups and other papers*. Tavistock.

Blau, B., & Siegel, E. V. (1978). Breathing together: A preliminary investigation of an involuntary reflex as adaptation. *American Journal of Dance Therapy, 2*(1), 35–42.

Bohleber, W. (2007). Remembrance, trauma, and collective memory: The battle for memory in psychoanalysis. *The International Journal of Psychoanalysis, 88*(2), 329–352. https://doi.org/10.1516/V5H5-8351-7636-7878

Boldt, G., & Pivnick, B. A. (2013). Moments of meeting: Learning to play with reading resistance. In M. O'Loughlin (Ed.), *The uses of psychoanalysis in working with children's lives* (pp. 245–263). Jason Aronson.

Boss, P. (2022). *The myth of closure: Ambiguous loss in a time of pandemic and change*. W. W. Norton.

Boulanger, G. (2011). *Wounded by reality: Understanding and treating adult onset trauma*. Routledge.

Brackett, B. M., & Cipriano, C. (2020, April 7). Teachers are anxious and overwhelmed. They need SEL now more than ever. *Ed Surge*. https://www.edsurge.com/news/2020-04-07-teachers-are-anxious-and-overwhelmed-they-need-sel-now-more-than-ever

Bragin, M., & Bragin, K. B. (2010). Making meaning together: Helping survivors of violence to learn at school. *Journal of Infant, Child, and Adolescent Psychotherapy, 9*(2–3), 47–67. https://doi.org/10.1080/15289168.2010.510986

Bromberg, P. (1998). *Standing in the spaces*. Psychology Press.

Caruth, C. (1996). *Unclaimed experience: Trauma, narrative, and history*. Johns Hopkins University Press.

Closson, T. (2023, June 20). Brooklyn school pioneers unified program to teach children with disabilities. *New York Times*, p. A 18.

Cohen, J. (2007). Interdisciplinary psychoanalysis and the education of children: Psychoanalytic and educational partnerships. *The Psychoanalytic Study of the Child, 62*, 180–207.

Cohen, J. (2014). Mental health clinicians and educators learning together: School climate reform and the promotion of effective K-12 risk prevention/health promotion efforts. *Journal of Infant, Child, and Adolescent Psychotherapy, 13*(4),342–349. https://doi.org/10.1080/15289168.2014.951273

Cohen, J., Espelage, D. L., Twemlow, S. W., Berkowitz, M. W., & Comer, J. P. (2015). Rethinking effective bully and violence prevention efforts: Promoting healthy school climates, positive youth development, and preventing bully-victim-by-stander behavior. *International Journal of Violence and schools, 15*(1), 2–40.

Cortina, M. (2024). Prologue: Erich Fromm's relevance for our troubled world. *Psychoanalytic Inquiry, 44*(1), 1–8. https://doi.org/10.1080/07351690.2024.2296336

Cushman, P. (1996). *Constructing the self, constructing America: A cultural history of psychotherapy*. DaCapo Press.

Cushman, P. (2015). Relational psychoanalysis as political resistance. *Contemporary Psychoanalysis, 51*(3), 423–459.

Dalal, F. (1998). *Taking the group seriously*. Jessica Kingsley Press.

Daniels, E. (2023). *The regulated classroom: "Bottom up" trauma-informed teaching*. Here This Now Publishing.

Danto, E. A. (2005). *Freud's free clinics: Psychoanalysis and social justice: 1918–1938*. Columbia University Press.

Davids, F. (2002). September 11th, 2001: Some thoughts on racism and religious prejudice as an obstacle. *British Journal of Psychotherapy, 18*(3), 361–366. https://doi.org/10.1111/j.1752-0118.2002.tb00037.x

Davids, F. (2011). *Internal racism: A psychoanalytic approach to race and difference*. Bloomsbury Publishing.

Davoine, F., & J. M. Gaudillière. (2005). *History beyond trauma: Whereof one cannot speak, thereof one cannot stay silent*. Other Press.

Dietrich, L. (2021). Higher expectations of teachers are not sufficient: How to take the next big step in social-emotional teacher training. *International Journal of Applied Psychoanalytic Studies, 18*(3), 319–329. https://doi.org/10.1002/aps.1724

Doerrfeld, C. (2018). *The rabbit listened*. Random.

Elbakoury, F. (2024, July 24). What I need from my White peers to thrive as a teacher of color. *EdSurge*. https://www.edsurge.com/news/2024-07-24-what-i-need-from-my-white-peers-to-thrive-as-a-teacher-of-color

Eng, D., & Han, S. (2000). A dialogue on racial melancholia. *Psychoanalytic Dialogues, 10*(4), 667–700. https://doi.org/10.1080/10481881009348576

Erikson, E. (1963). *Childhood and society* (2nd ed.). W. W. Norton.

Erikson, E.H. (1959). *Identity and the life cycle: Selected papers*. International Universities Press.

Erikson, E. H. (1968). *Identity, youth, and crisis* (No. 7). WW Norton & Company.

Erikson, E. H. (1994a). *Identity and the life cycle*. WW Norton & Company.

Erikson, E. H. (1994b). *Insight and responsibility: Lectures on the ethical implications of psychological insight*. WW Norton & Company.

Fonagy, P. (1991). Thinking about thinking: Some clinical and theoretical considerations in the treatment of a borderline patient. *International Journal of Psychoanalysis, 72*(4), 639–656.

Fonagy, P., Gergely, G., & Jurist, E. L. (Eds.). (2018). *Affect regulation, mentalization, and the development of the self*. Routledge.

Fonagy, P., Luyten, P., Allison, E., & Campbell, C. (2017). What we have changed our minds about: Part 1. Borderline personality disorder as a limitation of resilience. *Borderline Personality Disorder and Emotion Dysregulation, 4*(1), 11. https://doi.org/10.1186/s40479-017-0061-9

Forner, C. (2018). What mindfulness can learn about dissociation and what dissociation can learn from mindfulness. *Journal of Trauma & Dissociation, 20*(1), 1–15. https://doi.org/10.1080/15299732.2018.1502568

Frie, R., & Sauvayre, P. (Eds.). (2022). *Culture, politics, and race in the making of interpersonal psychoanalysis*. Routledge.

Gerson, S. (2009). When the third is dead: Memory, mourning, and witnessing in the aftermath of the Holocaust. *The International Journal of Psychoanalysis, 90*(6), 1341–1357. https://doi.org/10.1111/j.1745-8315.2009.00214.x

Glassman, U. (Ed.). (2008). *Group work: A humanistic and skills-building approach* (Vol. 13). SAGE Publications, Inc.

Gobodo-Madikizela, P. (2015). Psychological repair: The intersubjective dialogue of remorse and forgiveness in the aftermath of gross human rights violations. *Journal of the American Psychoanalytic Association, 63*(6), 1085–1123. https://doi.org/10.1177/0003065115615578

Gobodo-Madikizela, P. (2024). The time of *Nachträglichkeit* and the afterlife of apartheid trauma. *International Journal of Psychoanalysis, 105*(5):766–777. https://doi.org/10.1080/00207578.2024.2403235

González, F. J. (2020). Trump cards and Klein bottles: On the collective of the individual. *Psychoanalytic Dialogues, 30*(4), 383–398. https://doi.org/10.1080/10481885.2020.1774335

González, F. J., & Peltz, R. (2021). Community psychoanalysis: Collaborative practice as intervention. *Psychoanalytic Dialogues, 31*(4), 409–427. https://doi.org/10.1080/10481885.2021.1926788

Green, M. R., & Crowley, R. M. (1983). Revolution within psychoanalysis: A history of the William Alanson White Institute (Unpublished manuscript, 20 pp.).

Hagman, G. (2015). *Creative analysis: Art, creativity, and clinical process*. Routledge

Harris, A. (2019). From "What's American about American Psychoanalysis (2004)" to "What's American history and politics got to do with the emergence of the relational turn (2012) and on to the American Nightmare: 2017". *Psychoanalytic Inquiry*, 39(2), 138–145. https://doi.org/10.1080/07351690.2019.1561093

Hassinger, J., & Pivnick, B.A. (2021, October). The Psychoanalytic Community Collaboratory: A methodology for preparing practitioners to work in community spaces. *The Psychoanalytic Activist*. https://psychoanalyticactivist.com/2021/10/04/the-psychoanalytic-community-collaboratory-a-methodology-for-preparing-practitioners-to-work-in-community-spaces/

Hassinger, J. A., & Pivnick, B.A. (2022). The "community turn": Relational citizenship in the Psychoanalytic Community Collaboratory. *International Journal of Psychoanalysis*, *103*(1), 120–143. https://doi.org/10.1080/00207578.2021.2017780

Hassinger, J. A., & Pivnick, B. A. (2024, September 2). "The 21st Century Psychoanalyst: Clinician, Community Member and Relational Citizen." Invited Talk. W.A. White Society Colloquium. William Alanson White Institute, New York City.

Hernández-Tubert, R. (2011). The politics of despair: From despair to dialogue and hope. *Group Analysis*, *44*(1), 27–39. https://doi.org/10.1177/0533316410390455

Holmes, D. (2016). "Culturally-imposed Trauma: The sleeping dog has awakened: Will psychoanalysis take heed?" *Psychoanalytic Dialogues*, *26*, 6, 641–654.

Hopper, E. (2003). *Traumatic experience in the unconscious life of groups*. Jessica Kingsley.

Hopper, E. (2009). The theory of the basic assumption of incohesion: Aggregation/massification or (BA) I:A/M. *British Journal of Psychotherapy*, *25*, 214–229.

Hopper, E., & Weinberg, H. (2011). *The social unconscious in persons, groups, and societies* (Vol 1: Mainly theory). Karnac Books.

Jose, C. (2024, May 1). Social-emotional learning strategies don't work for every student. Here's what does. *EdSurge Newsletter*, May 1, 2024.

Kabasakalian-McKay, R., & Mark, D. (Eds.). (2023). *Inhabiting implication in racial oppression and relational psychoanalysis*. Routledge.

Khetan, N. (2025, August 20). What I've learned about building citizens, not just students. *EdSurge*. https://www.edsurge.com/news/2025-08-20-what-i-ve-learned-about-building-citizens-not-just-students

Kliman, G. (2018). Reflective network therapy for childhood autism and childhood PTSD. *Neuropsychoanalysis*, *20*(2), 73–86. https://doi.org/10.1080/15294145.2018.1535279

Layton, L. (2013). Psychoanalysis and politics: Historicising subjectivity. *Mens Sana Monographs*, *11*(1), 68–81.

Layton, L. (2020). *Toward a social psychoanalysis: Culture, character, and normative unconscious processes*. Routledge.

Makari, G. (2008). *Revolution in mind: The creation of psychoanalysis – A groundbreaking history of the intellectual endeavor that transformed twentieth century thought*. Harper-Collins.

Menashe-Grinberg, A., Shneor, S., Meiri, G., & Atzaba-Poria, N. (2022). Improving the parent–child relationship and child adjustment through parental reflective functioning group intervention, *Attachment & Human Development*, *24*(2), 208–228. https://doi.org/10.1080/14616734.2021.1919159

Nardone, M., & Casado-Frankel, T. (2025). Managing the psychological aspects of deportation and child custody. *The Appleseed Network*. https://appleseednetwork.org/wp-content/uploads/2025/07/2025-Deportation-Preparation-Manual-for-Immigrant-Families-updated-7.8.25.pdf

New York City Department of Education. (2022). OPEN ARMS families seeking asylum: Comprehensive support plan NYC DOE. https://www.nyc.gov/content/dam/nycgov/mayors-office/downloads/pdf/press-releases/2022/OpenArms-Families-Seeking-Asylum.pdf

O'Loughlin, M. (Ed.) (2014). *The Ethics of Remembering and the Consequences of Forgetting: Essays on Trauma, History and Memory*. Rowman & Littlefield.

Ogden, T. (1994). *Subjects of analysis*. Routledge.

Pivnick, B. & Reading, R. (Co-hosts) (2024, November 21). Group psychology: The promise and perils of togetherness. *[Audio podcast episode]. In Couched.* https://couchedpodcast.org/group-psychology-the-promise-and-perils-of-togetherness/

Pivnick, B.A. (2011, September). Enacting remembrance: Turning toward memorializing September 11th. *Journal of Religion and Health*, *50*(3), 499–515. New York: Springer.

Pivnick, B. A. (2013). The beholder's share: An intersubjective review of Bromberg's *Shadow of the Tsunami. The Psychoanalytic Quarterly*, *82*(1), 179–192. https://doi.org/10.1002/j.2167-4086.2013.00017.x

Pivnick, B. A. (2015). Spaces to Stand in: Applying Clinical Psychoanalysis to the Relational Design of the National September 11 Memorial Museum. (Winner of the APA Division 39 Section Five Schillinger Memorial Essay Award.). *Division/Review*, *13*, 19–24.

Pivnick, B. A. (2017a). Creative analysis: Art, creativity, and clinical process by George Hagman. *The Psychoanalytic Quarterly*, *86*, 2, 508–513.

Pivnick, B. A. (2017b). Transforming collapse: Applying clinical psychoanalysis to the relational design of the National September 11 Memorial Museum. *International Forum of Psychoanalysis* (Violence, Terror and Terrorism Today: Psychoanalytic Perspectives, Part II), *26*(4), 248–257.

Pivnick, B. A. (2021). Recollecting the vanishing forms of 9/11: Twenty years of ruptures, ripples, and reflections. *Psychoanalytic Perspectives*, *18*(3), 279–295. https://doi.org/10.1080/1551806X.2021.1953874

Pivnick, B. A., & Hassinger, J. A. (2021). The child in the school, the school in the community, and the community in the child: Linking psychic and social domains in school violence prevention. *International Journal Applied Psychoanalytic Studies, 18*(1), 1–12. https://doi.org/10.1002/aps.1722

Pivnick, B. A., & Hassinger, J. A. (2022). The relational citizen as implicated subject: Emergent unconscious processes in the Psychoanalytic Community Collaboratory. In R. Kabasakalian-McKay & D. Mark (Eds.), *Inhabiting implication in racial oppression and relational psychoanalysis* (pp. 158–182). Routledge.

Pivnick, B. A., & Hassinger, J. A. (2026). The work and play of democracy: Growing relational citizens. *International Journal of Applied Psychoanalytic Studies, 23*(2), 1–14. https://doi.org/10.1002/aps.70043

Pivnick, B. A., & Hennes, T. (2014). Managing collapse: Memorializing September 11th through the co-creation of a memorial museum. In M. O'Loughlin (Ed.), *The ethics of remembering and the consequences of forgetting: Essays on trauma, history and memory* (pp. 325–354). Rowman & Littlefield.

Porges, S. (2011). *The polyvagal theory: Neurophysiological foundations of emotions, attachment, communication, and self-regulation*. W. W. Norton.

Pothireddy, K. (2024, September 25). Supporting young students' social emotional needs in the post-Covid era. *EdSurge*. https://www.edsurge.com/news/2024-09-25-supporting-young-students-social-emotional-needs-in-the-post-covid-era

Rothberg, M. (2019). *The implicated subject: Beyond victims and perpetrators*. Stanford University Press.

Rudden, M. G., & Twemlow, S. W. (2013). A beginning theory of action for community analysts based on group observation, theories of the unconscious, and evolutionary psychology. *International Journal of Applied Psychoanalytic Studies, 10*(3), 199–209. https://doi.org/10.1002/aps.1367

Salberg, J., & Grand, S. (Eds.). (2016). *Wounds of history: Repair and resilience in the trans-generational transmission of trauma*. Routledge.

Shapiro, E. R. (2019). *Finding a place to stand: Developing self-reflective institutions, leaders and citizens*. Phoenix Publishing House.

Shapiro, E. R., & Carr, A. W. (1991). *Lost in familiar places: Creating new connections between the individual and society*. Yale University Press.

Skaalvik, E. M., & Skaalvik, S. (2010). Teacher self-efficacy and teacher burnout: A study of relations. *Teaching and Teacher Education, 26*(4), 1059–1069. https://doi.org/10.1016/j.tate.2009.11.001

Sklarew, B., Twemlow, S., & Wilkinson, S. M. (2004). *Analysis in the trenches: Streets, schools, war zones*. Routledge.

Steele, H., & Steele, M. (2018). *Handbook of attachment-based interventions*. Guilford Publications.

Stephens, M. (2022). More simply human than otherwise: Interpersonal psychoanalysis and the field of the "Negro Problem". In R. Frie & P. Sauvayre (Eds.), *Culture, politics and race in the making of interpersonal psychoanalysis*. Routledge.

Stern, D. B. (2010). *Partners in thought: Working with unformulated experience, dissociation, and enactment*. Routledge.

Stern, D. B. (2015). *Relational freedom: Emergent properties of the interpersonal field*. Routledge.

Stern, D. B. (2023). *On coming into possession of oneself: Transformations of the interpersonal field*. Routledge.

Sullivan, H. S. (1953/1968). *The interpersonal theory of psychiatry*. Norton.

Switchboard. (2023, June 21). Traumatic stress among refugee children and youth. Part one: Viewing trauma through a developmental lens. https://www.switchboardta.org/resource/traumatic-stress-among-refugee-children-and-youth-part-i-viewing-trauma-through-a-developmental-lens/

Switchboard. (2024, March 29). The eight stages of co-creation: Tips for refugee service providers on using inclusive approaches in their work. https://www.switchboardta.org/the-eight-stages-of-co-creation-tips-for-refugee-service-providers-on-using-inclusive-approaches-in-their-work/

Thapa, A., Cohen, J., Higgins-D'Alessandro, A., & Guffey, S. (2013). A review of school climate research. *Review of Educational Research*, *83*, 3, 357–385. https://doi.org/10.3102/0034654313483907

Tubert-Oklander, J. (2014). *The one and the many: Relational psychoanalysis and group analysis*. Routledge.

Tubert-Oklander, J., & Hernández de Tubert, R. (2004). *Operative groups: The Latin-American approach to group analysis* (Vol. 24). Jessica Kingsley Publishers.

Tubert-Oklander, J., & Hernández-Tubert, R. (2021). *Psychoanalysis, group analysis, and beyond: Towards a new paradigm of the human being*. Routledge.

Twemlow, S., & Parens, H. (2006). Might Freud's legacy lie beyond the couch? *Psychoanalytic Psychology*, *23*(2), 430–451. https://doi.org/10.1037/0736-9735.23.2.430

Vaughans, K. (2016). To unchain haunting blood memories. In J. Salberg & S. Grand (Eds.), *Wounds of history. Repair and resilience in the transgenerational transmission of trauma* (pp. 226–239). Routledge.

Volkan, V. D. (2013). Large-group-psychology in its own right: Large-group identity and peace making. *International Journal of Applied Psychoanalytic Studies*, *10*(3), 210–246. https://doi.org/10.1002/aps.1368

Will, M. (2022 June 15). Paraprofessionals: As the "backbones" of the classroom, they get low pay, little support. *Education Week*. https://www.edweek.org/leadership/paraprofessionals-as-the-backbones-of-the-classroom-they-get-low-pay-little-support/2022/06

Wyatt, R., & Beznes, A. (2026). Beyond borders: Psychoanalytic perspectives on refugee healing. In J. Dobrich (Ed.), *Moving from grievance to hope in psychoanalysis: Applied case studies*. Routledge, this volume.

Chapter 8

Ethnocultural Identity and Attachment

Unraveling Legacies of Self-Erasure

Johanna Dobrich

> Education is the first form of activism—but to educate others, we must first educate ourselves.
>
> (Freeman, 2021, p. 97)

Introduction

This chapter examines how a contemporary developmental psychoanalytic framework can illuminate the impact of, and ameliorate responses to, inherited cultural shame and internalized bias. I argue that *internalized* self-alienation, manifesting as internalized racism, antisemitism, sexism, homophobia, xenophobia, and similar identity-based biases, can be understood as complex, often unconscious responses stemming from insecure or disorganized relational dynamics between marginalized groups and the dominant[1] culture. These responses appear as split-off aspects within a complex and evolving identity shaped by systemic oppression and resilience, aspects of self that influence the whole from beneath awareness, often without being easily noticed or transformed. Among marginalized peoples, the unconscious incorporation of negative or distorted projections from those who hold cultural power and security is not a new phenomenon. It is ancient and well-documented across anthropological studies of oppressed and disempowered groups. The pernicious impact of internalizing the hate, bias, and indifference of others reinforces dissociation, disempowerment, and, ultimately, grievance.

As this collection of essays aims to address, it is not a simple task to move out of states of chronic grievance and into *intersubjective relationality*. Supporting the vulnerability inherent in complexity and exposure

DOI: 10.4324/9781003658382-9

requires both individual effort and systemic structures that respond with genuine recognition.[2] The path toward integrative cultural self-reclamation among disempowered and/or marginalized peoples involves fostering a sense of security by transforming internalized projections that exist both *within* individuals and in the broader social context, alongside collective efforts toward social inclusion and relational recognition. "Coming out" or "coming home" to oneself and consolidating self-pride within one's marginalized communities of origin, *while also* maintaining the capacity to relate across difference and move beyond one's own ethnocultural borders, is a necessary foundation for intersubjective relating in a *pluralist model*.[3] In the process of maturing toward pluralism and intersubjectivity, marginalized peoples face the profound challenge of transmuting deeply held emotions elicited from their objectification such as anger and envy, while cultivating the capacity for connection. This emotional work is essential to making space for both the self and the "Other" in relinquishing internalized projections. Given that these dynamics often span generations, there is also the critical task of disidentifying from caretakers who themselves may carry these projections, a process that involves living with the self-alienation and deprecation that arise from intergenerational racial melancholia and dissociation (Eng & Han, 2019). Relational healing is an intergenerational, multilayered process.

Pluralism then includes both the plurality of internal relations among one's *intra-identifications* and multiple external relations between individuals, peoples, and groups. The maintenance of split or dissociated identifications between one's Otherness and one's relation to dominant cultural ideologies may keep people inadvertently locked into states of grievance, where their own and the Others' recognition becomes severely impaired, leaving them vulnerable to repetitive reenactments of power and powerlessness, extremist "solutions,"[4] and unintegrated actions. For example, Fanon explores the concept of doubling primarily in *Black Skin, White Masks* (1952/2008), describing it as a psychological experience in which racially oppressed individuals develop a split consciousness, caught between their own sense of self and the ways they are perceived or defined by the dominant oppressive culture. In this dynamic, experiences of victimization can become embedded in self-identity, reinforcing bonds with caretakers who themselves carry the weight of marginalization. This is not to deny the reality of actual victimization experienced by those marginalized but to underscore its profound psychological imprint on how we organize our sense of self.

Moving from the rigidity of defense to the openness of a fluid conversation transforms the way one experiences their identities (Hart, 2017). Stephens (2020) describes the deeply human tension that arises in intersubjective life as the psychic labor of holding our own self-perception *alongside* the images reflected back by another. This is not simply about being seen but about enduring the complexity of *being seen differently than we see ourselves*, without losing sight of self-possession, as the work of perception is always a fluid, multidimensional field. Intersubjective relational life requires cultivating the capacity to metabolize the Other's gaze without forfeiting one's own, a task that is as developmental as it is existential and often charged with historical, cultural, and affective weight. Metabolization is not the same as unconscious identification. Metabolization, also called *mentalization*, involves the capacity to reflect on and make sense of emotional experiences (Fonagy et al., 2002). Introjection, by contrast, is a reactive process rooted in early attachment relationships, in which a child unconsciously absorbs messages and emotions from a threatening or inconsistent relational environment without conscious thought or understanding (Benjamin, 1995; Harris, 2009; Mitchell, 2000). When cultural biases that generate self-hatred, self-alienation, and despair are introjected, they disrupt the ongoing development of intersubjective capacities, shaping how individuals relate to themselves and to others within the social field.

Individual psychoanalysts have a vital role to play in bringing the tensions between *being seen* and *being oneself* into conscious awareness, at the personal, professional, and social levels, teaching people how to shift their self-concept from one rooted in adaptation, insecurity, and defense to one grounded in self-sovereignty and a capacity for intercultural connection. Anton Hart (2017) writes,

> When it comes to the problem of prejudice, psychoanalysis offers a more profound remedy than trying to teach people not to be prejudiced or to watch what they say. Because psychoanalysis is interested in understanding what would make one person hate another and is inherently interested in creating contained opportunities for

> dialogue. Psychoanalysis aspires to help people to become more aware of the ways ignorance is self-protective and that prejudice involves using people to manage dreaded internal experience.
>
> (pp. 17–20)

It is through such dialogue that our automated defensive responses may change.

Ethnocultural Identity as an Attachment-Based Experience

What mechanisms account for the incorporation of bias when on the conscious level it seems self-defeating to take in these kinds of adverse appraisals? Why are marginalized individuals particularly vulnerable to harmful, neglectful, or distorting narratives about their communal identity? Sociology, anthropology, and psychology each offer distinct vantage points for understanding how *structural self-dispossession* shape's identity: sociology highlights unequal systems of power and exclusion; anthropology attends to cultural dislocation and the loss of collective meaning; whereas psychology examines the impact of early interpersonal environments. Contemporary psychoanalysis adds another layer of understanding—a developmental lens, particularly through attachment theory, that helps us understand how internalized bias can emerge not only within the individual psyche but also through *collective cultural transmissions*. The "telescoping"[5] of generational traumas, as well as the range of possible defensive adaptations that accompany them, goes beyond the individual family story and is carried by *ethno-collective narratives* about identity and power (Faimberg, 1988). In the context of social marginalization, negative cultural messages can be incorporated pre-reflectively, shaping self-concept through external devaluation and driving defensive strategies often misread as "choices" that function to protect both physical and psychological safety at the group level.[6] For example, comedians frequently draw attention to ethno-racial stereotypes associated with different socio-ethnic groups; yet underlying the humor is an implicit recognition that these cultural "traits" and archetypes often represent collective adaptations to intergenerational patterns of insecure attachment and unresolved dynamics of power and marginalization.[7]

For example, Stoute's (2019) work offers a psychoanalytic lens through which racial identity is understood as a culturally transmitted construct, not merely a personal one. She emphasizes how societal messages about race are unconsciously passed down across generations, shaping internal psychic structures as they become a part of the cultural identity. These inherited narratives can sustain bias and emotional wounding, ultimately disrupting mentalization and undermining the development of a stable and integrated self-concept, as well as any room for the concept of the "Other." Even in the absence of overt abuse or hostility, messages of inferiority can be subtly transmitted intergenerationally. When communities themselves have internalized societal bias, they may consciously and unconsciously pass on messages of caution, silence, or disidentification as protective strategies to kin, further reinforcing the internalization of bias. From a contemporary Freudian lens, Apprey (2023) examines how historical wounds of racism, oppression, and domination endured by collective identities often reemerge disguised in the present as dislocated, mystifying symptoms within individuals, using psychoanalysis to transform and relieve people of these "toxic errands" and "haunts." To this end, Echegoyen (2022) emphasizes that psychoanalysis should not only focus on individual intrapsychic processes but also consider how racism operates in the relational and societal fields, influencing identity formation and internalized oppression. Racism is not simply internalized; it is experienced and negotiated across relationships and social structures, perpetuating a recursive loop that shapes both self and social reality.

Contemporary psychoanalysis highlights the vital role of the "witness," a relational stance held in the space between experiences of power and powerlessness. Intrapersonally, the witnessing function registers and holds the impact of events on one's sense of self, creating an internal "third" capable of integrating conflicting experiences, as described by Bromberg, Stern, Gerson, and others. This third can extend beyond the individual, forming the basis for witnessing communities. Crucially, the witness must operate on multiple levels: within the psyche of the marginalized individual, within the therapeutic dyad between analyst and patient, and, as this chapter illustrates, within the broader social space where communities engage and interact.

Social media, journalism, and communal discourse serve as cultural sites for the witnessing community, or its absence, where experiences of human struggle and bias are made visible or rendered mute. The absence of a witnessing community, combined with the frequent overrepresentation of internalized *isms* in mainstream cultural discourse, deepens self-alienation among the marginalized. Echegoyen (2022) extends this understanding of active engagement through the concept of community psychoanalysis, which moves beyond the individual to address the collective and relational dimensions of identity and oppression. By situating psychoanalytic work within social and cultural contexts, this approach facilitates shared reflection and healing around systemic racism and internalized oppression experienced by different groups and communities.[8]

Extending attachment theory's insights about the effects of disorganized and insecure relational bonds on the psyche and self-concept to the collective domain offers a deeper understanding of how culturally marginalized individuals may come to internalize dominant cultural projections and biases. This internalization is especially likely in the absence of an attuned "third" who can provide security and help foster a coherent sense of self. In the absence of a witnessing community, individuals may be left psychologically undefended. The deeply ingrained human need for attachment often comes at the cost of self-cohesion, creating profound psychic lacerations.

I am not speaking here of the broader psychological goal of "belonging." Rather, attachment provides the developmental and psychodynamic foundation upon which the capacity for belonging and recognition later rests. When we extend our understanding of insecure attachment dynamics to the level of culture, we can observe parallel patterns among marginalized communities that resemble the experiences of infants raised by caregivers who are unavailable or unsafe. Communities, particularly those shaped by histories of collective trauma, marginalization, and systemic violence, may internalize a fractured or conditional sense of attachment. If the host culture or dominant social structure is both a symbolic caregiver (offering protection, resources, and identity) and a source of danger (through exclusion, surveillance, derision, or oppression), this creates a kind of collective disorganized attachment. In this relational context, we often see signs of chronic mistrust, difficulties with collective identification, internalized oppression, and cycles of projection and scapegoating. The very institutions meant to provide safety (i.e., government, healthcare, education, and law enforcement) become unsafe or rejecting. Just like the infant with a disorganized attachment style, the community oscillates between seeking connection and fearing/encountering annihilation and betrayal from their "scaregivers"[9] (Epstein, 2018).

Without a scaffold to develop secure early attachments between a marginalized group and their host culture, the psyche may struggle to tolerate difference, seek inclusion, or internalize recognition from others. The psychological strengths and constraints conferred by group belonging, such as identity coherence and collective resilience, may be weakened when the group's relationship to the dominant culture is shaped by disorganized or insecure attachment. In such cases, any intragroup identifications will also carry internalized shame, mistrust, and defensive distancing that constrains the transformative potential held within belonging. What gets forsaken may be a space in which to balance the need for belonging to a cultural group, with the need for autonomy, individuality, recognition, and difference.

An insecure or disorganized attachment system requires individuals to adapt to others' needs at the expense of their authentic selves in order to maintain the asymmetrical relationship. The quality of the relationship is not what matters at the earliest of levels, just that it be there, so as to avoid encountering the primitive agonies Winnicott outlined so long ago, of an immature ego alone in the world. Children do not have a choice about whether to abide by this; they simply accommodate the conditions set by their caregivers to keep the connection. Similarly, citizens, while not children, are positioned to depend on governments and political structures to sustain essential security and care within the social field.

So, attachment works at the level of culture too. We form an attachment bond to the place, space, time, and region in which we grow and live.[10] Belonging is a powerful psychological motive that drives relational development[11] (Freud, 1931; Fromm, 1956). One way of recognizing racial-socioeconomic privilege is to see it as a secure attachment between a people and their host culture. It is no small thing to have a secure attachment between one's sociocultural identity and the host culture. Secure attachments provide emotional safety and alignment between one's identity and the wider field, mirroring self-concepts back with ease, an effective context that supports emotional expression, regulation, shared normative values and goals, the presence of strong interpersonal relationships, resilience to stress, and the confidence to explore and enjoy one's sovereignty, while remaining connected to something greater. Viewing the relationship between marginalized identities and a host culture through an attachment lens not only reveals how attachment dynamics operate across the social field but also identifies points where intervention can support connection, security, and integration.

Acculturation Strategies, Defenses, and Attachment

The social psychologist John Berry highlights how different acculturation strategies impact psychological well-being, social adjustment, and identity development. Berry's (1997) model outlines four different strategies minority communities may adopt in response to cultural contact with a dominant society. I am adding in a trauma-informed framework identifying the *dynamic defenses* at play in each strategy. Berry's model includes four possible pathways: **assimilation**, where individuals abandon their original culture in favor of the dominant one; **integration**, where both the original and dominant cultures are maintained; **separation**, where individuals retain their original culture while rejecting the dominant culture; and **marginalization**, where both the original and dominant cultures are rejected. This framework helps to explain the varied ways individuals and communities navigate a specific cultural identity within the context of their attachment to their host culture (Table 8.1).

A psychoanalytic lens, however, reveals that these pathways are not selected consciously but rather grow out of attachment styles and the defenses they mobilize. A secure cultural attachment would promote a degree of integration between a marginalized group and their host culture; whereas insecure and disorganized attachments would lend themselves to defensive postures such as *assimilation*, where one's authentic cultural heritage is diluted, diminished, or erased; *separation*, where one remains entrenched in their ethnocultural identity but remains impervious to modifying or being influenced by anything outside it; and *marginalization*, where a person's cultural identity is caught, never becoming

Table 8.1 Berry's Acculturation Strategies as Seen Through the Lens of Attachment and Defense

Berry's Acculturation Strategy	*Description*	*Common Trauma Defenses*	*Predominant Attachment Style*	*Psychological and Relational Implications*
Assimilation	Adopting the host culture while rejecting the original culture	Denial, suppression of original identity, **Flight/Fawn**	Insecure: Anxious-preoccupied or dismissive	Internal conflict, loss of cultural self, possible alienation from original community, inhibited mentalization of "self" but knowledge of "other"
Separation	Maintaining original culture and rejecting the host culture	Avoidance, withdrawal, splitting, **Fight**	Insecure: Avoidant or disorganized	Cultural protection may feel safe, but isolation and rigidity may maintain trauma responses, inhibited mentalization of "other"
Marginalization	Losing connection to both cultures	Dissociation, fragmentation **Freeze**	Insecure: Disorganized	High risk for identity confusion, isolation, and unresolved trauma
Integration	Maintaining and accessing both original and new cultures	Flexible defenses, cohesive identity	Secure or moving toward *earned* security	Greater psychological flexibility, resilience, and identity coherence, mentalization of self/ other, intersubjective relationality

Note: The author offers a perspective that integrates a trauma-informed, attachment-focused lens with Berry's established acculturation categories by adding in the attachment classification and the psychological/relational implications.

assimilated nor remaining authentically connected to one's heritage, a liminal space of nonbeing between worlds defined by dissociative absence and melancholia.[12] If we consider these cultural pathways not as consciously chosen identities but as expressions shaped by early attachment experiences, what shifts in our understanding? What becomes possible if we view cultural positioning as, in part, an unconscious strategy to manage relational safety and vulnerability? And what role might psychoanalysis play in addressing these developmental attachment wounds not just within the individual but at the level of the social?

A Case Study: Tackling Jewish Self-Erasure in the American Diaspora Post-10/7

In the sections that follow, I explore the relationship between enculturation and intersubjective development through the lens of attachment within culturally situated marginalized identities using a case example.[13] I use anti-Jewish bias in the North American Jewish diaspora to illustrate how disorganized attachment can operate in this framework, shaping the self through the introjection of disavowal, distortion, and cultural rejection. I then describe a clinical community-based project aimed at addressing internalized anti-Jewish bias as one model of applied contemporary psychoanalytic action. In today's cultural and political climate, the marginalization of Jews as an ethnocultural identity is overlooked, politicized, and misunderstood, making the task of addressing antisemitism both urgent and psychologically complex (Erlich, 2025).[14] This complexity only deepens when antisemitism is strategically deployed as a political tool to justify oppressive actions of contemporary nation states, further distorting its meaning and eroding the possibility for sincere engagement. From a psychoanalytic perspective, antisemitism operates not only as a social and political force but also as a psychic one, embedded in collective unconscious narratives, disavowed projections, and historical trauma (Erlich, 2025). This chapter attends to *internalized* antisemitism as a form of "othering" that often operates invisibly within both cultural discourse and individual subjectivity. To examine internalized antisemitism through a psychoanalytic lens is to explore how it is enacted and transmitted both intergenerationally and intrapsychically and to consider how it functions as a defense against deeper anxieties about power, difference, belonging, and connection—the bedrocks of relational life. Despite the specificity of the case example, my hope is that the model offered provides a resonant framework for understanding the psychic impact of marginalization across a range of cultural and collective identities.

Like other minority-immigrant groups, Jewish people have experienced a disorganized attachment to their host cultures, shaped by centuries of exile, bias, and scapegoating, reflecting the persistent and shape-shifting nature of antisemitism in every place they have lived (Erlich, 2025). Similar to other marginalized groups who face racial triangulation, long-standing anti-Jewish bias has resulted not only in episodes of violence and death but also in systemic discrimination, exclusion, and stereotyping. For example, Asian Americans frequently experience racial triangulation within the Black-White framework of American society, while Jewish Americans often occupy a similarly ambiguous racial position, seen as either "too White" or "not White enough," even though Jews do not self-define along racial lines and represent a plurality of races (Freeman, 2021; Kim, 1999). Jewish ethnic identity emerges from a history that both predates and resists reduction to the categories of race that structure American life, complicating straightforward narratives of racialization. The experience of belonging to a minority group marked by both historical marginalization and generational erasure, yet also rich with internal diversity and resiliencies, creates ongoing struggles around inclusion, exclusion, and recognition both between people *within* the group and in the larger social context.[15]

Jewish identity transcends religiosity, functioning as a civilization or "peoplehood" (Freeman, 2021). Thus, one need not be religious to experience the damaging effects of antisemitism on self-identity and self-concept. Jews face a persistent double bind imposed by their host cultures (the attachment figure): either fully assimilate and give up authentic identity to gain social security or maintain their distinctiveness and endure exclusion, bias, and derision.[16] How individual Jews navigate this tension varies, shaped by intergenerational inheritance, family circumstances, and geography. Many reconcile the double bind imposed by the epigenic response to historical persecution unconsciously (Felsen, 2017). Some lean toward assimilation to minimize any felt sense of risk and to fit in (*fawn*), others preserve a primary Jewish identity and minimize or diminish investment outside the community (*fight*), and many remain in a state of *freeze*, identifying as "Jew-*ish*," without actively integrating the particular identity or the broader culture.[17] Identity integration requires a foundational sense of attachment security to meaningfully engage with the enduring legacies of hatred (i.e., how one is hated, how one may come to hate others, and how self-hatred can take root), approaching these dynamics with consciousness, care, and curiosity (Pogue-White, 2002). But these difficult truths often trigger defensive shutdowns that block reflection and dialogue, both within individuals and across communities.

The events of October 7 shattered a sense of psychic safety within and across the Jewish diaspora, reactivating generational trauma tied to persecution, exile, and collective vulnerability (Felsen, 2017, 2021). The attack ruptured deeply held assumptions about protection and belonging, triggering feelings of helplessness, hypervigilance, and profound dislocation. For many, it evoked unconscious fears of annihilation and abandonment, echoes of historical trauma encoded in both individual and communal memory. The result was not only disenfranchised grief, outrage, and fear but also a destabilizing loss of symbolic containment, leaving many diaspora Jews struggling to reestablish a coherent narrative of personal identity and safety in the world. The shattering of safety, inclusion, and acceptance is not a new phenomenon for Jewish communities. As a result, decisions about carrying one's Jewishness are often shaped unconsciously in response to external pressures rather than through inward reflection and choice (Pogue-White, 2002). Of course, there are those who struggle and manage to integrate their Jewish identity within their American identity despite the complications of historical traumas and legacies. But many struggle to have the psychic space and capacity to do so in an environment permeated by legacies of persecution and discrimination and active ruptures in the present tense. How can one experience recognition or engage in true intersubjective relating when they are caught in patterns of self-erasure and defense?

Freeman (2021) elaborates on the historical precedent of Jewish people being forced to fundamentally alter their identities to accommodate the non-Jewish world's distorted perceptions of who they are.[18] Psychologically, it may be more accurate to say that this survival response is inherited rather than consciously chosen. Gilman (1985) observes that the identity fragmentation resulting from this double bind often leads to the unconscious emergence of self-hatred.

This turning against oneself to survive is not a new phenomenon. W.E.B. Du Bois (1903) first articulated the concept of double consciousness to describe the internal conflict experienced by Black individuals navigating a White-supremacist society, shaped by the legacy of slavery and systemic racism and the resulting insecure attachment to the host culture. Similarly, Jewish people have carried a form of double consciousness shaped by their long history as an exiled minority subjected to violence and persecution over millennia, alongside a legacy of survival and achievement. This double consciousness creates a vulnerability to projection that a more integrated self-awareness might better defend against. The consequence is a heightened incidence of unconscious self-alienation and self-hatred. Pogue-White (2002) argues that effectively addressing racial hatred requires acknowledging all three dimensions of hate: not only how we are hated, or how we hate others, but also *how we hate ourselves*.

Internalized self-hatred functions unconsciously to protect us from feeling exposed, powerless, or profoundly alone. It emerges in contexts where rejection, threat, or shame have become woven into our sense of self, in relation to our cultural and communal identities. But that protection comes at a steep cost: it fractures our self-worth, disrupts a coherent sense of identity, and limits our capacity for relational intimacy. We become estranged not only from others but also from ourselves. In individual treatment, part of the therapeutic task is to trace how disavowed defensive operations, and the parts of the self they protect, came to be internalized, and to name the shame, disenfranchisement, and grief around cultural identity that was never truly one's to carry. Social psychoanalysis has a role to play in this process. When we understand the psychic function of this hatred, we can begin to gently externalize it, to grieve what was lost in its formation, and to slowly reintegrate acceptance for parts of ourselves that had to go into hiding with tenderness, with dignity, and with greater choice moving forward.

Internalized Antisemitism: The Hidden Wounds of Disorganized Attachment

The intrapsychic and structural components of internalized antisemitism function like other defenses: they protect the self by reducing complexity and relocating what is frightening in the external world back inside the individual. Self-hatred and its subtler counterpart, self-erasure, offer a powerful, protective response to being targeted and marginalized by dominant groups. *Now you see it, now you don't.* Internalized antisemitism is thus transmitted intergenerationally through attachment systems, both at the cultural level and within individual families. It involves an automatic response to perceived and actual threats within the context of cultural attachment, and it is better understood as occurring at subliminal levels rather than as a consciously adopted identification with the aggressor.

Fortunately, Jewish communities, like other marginalized groups, possess rich cultural strengths that include a commitment to education and the pursuit of knowledge, *chavruta* (the study of texts in pairs or groups), communal caregiving networks, tradition, historicity, an openness to interpretation and debate, language and ritual, celebration of pluralism, *tikkun olam* (repairing the world), and an emphasis on *chesed* (kindness), to name a few. This tapestry of resiliencies is also transmitted through the attachment system. However, unlike other marginalized groups, Jews are less likely to have allies *outside their own* communities within progressive, multicultural, and social justice spaces to help amplify these resiliencies, making the burden of internalized antisemitism a particularly potent force for defenses such as self-erasure and cultural alienation[19] (Freeman, 2021). In the absence of consistent and clear allyship, resiliencies may become increasingly difficult to sustain and transmit intergenerationally, as defensive survival strategies can give rise to modes of acculturation that ultimately constrain access to these very forms of resilience. As Freeman (2021) writes, "Jewish pride asserts our Jewishness as an equal partner to our other identities while refusing to subvert it for acceptance" (p. 122). However, this stance is not equally accessible to all; for many, it must be arduously attained through what is known as "earned secure attachment"[20] (Roisman et al., 2002). A secure racial identity grows in the presence of relationships and communities that witness and affirm one's experience altering intrapsychic templates. These moments of recognition allow resilience to take root. Over time, they shape a coherent, embodied sense of self that carries one through the challenges of the world with both agency and openness.

Moving beyond grievance and defensive strategies toward communal sovereignty, connection, and hope in this context involves the challenging process of working through internalized antisemitism and transcending inherited defensive structures that contribute to self-erasure. Communal sovereignty here refers to the collective empowerment and self-determination of the community, reclaiming agency over its identity, cultural practices, and narratives in the face of extremist external pressures and historical oppression. This process enables a restoration of communal integrity and resilience, fostering authentic connection and the possibility of intersubjective relating. This transformation takes place within a social and historical reality in which Jewish existence has been threatened not only by dominant cultures but also by other marginalized groups, whether passively through acculturation pressures or actively through persecution and exclusion. For example, Bar-Halpern and Wolfman (2025) explore how traumatic invalidation experienced by many diaspora Jews has only intensified the psychological impact of the October 7 attacks among North American Jews and within the mental health professions in particular. They examine how responses of denial, blame, and emotional neglect across personal, institutional, and societal levels have compounded the intergenerational trauma held within the Jewish community. Their work highlights how invalidation at the social level disrupts self-perception, emotional regulation, and worldview. What constitutes secure attachment for Jewish individuals remains an underexplored question within psychoanalytic literature, as this area is not typically considered relevant to the study of marginalization and identity politics. Rather than offering models of individuals who confront and transform their internalized antisemitism, psychoanalysis has more frequently depicted its enactment, often without any critical reflection or repair.

Moreover, contemporary literature on internalized homophobia and racism often unintentionally reinforces antisemitism by portraying Jewish founders of psychoanalysis as privileged White colonizers, overlooking their lived experience as members of a minority culture subject to persecution and attempted erasure.[21] The Nazi regime's systematic suppression of psychoanalysis through targeting its Jewish practitioners and institutions underscores this history. For instance, the Berlin Psychoanalytic Institute's Jewish leadership was forcibly removed and replaced by a non-Jewish director to align with Nazi ideology (Ellenberger, 1970; Frosh, 2005). This action was part of a broader campaign to erase psychoanalysis as a so-called Jewish science under the Third Reich, a painful chapter in the field's communal legacy (Frosh, 2005; Laub, 1992). Today, Jewish identity risks being flattened into simplistic labels like "oppressor" or "privileged," erasing the structural realities of anti-Jewish bias and reflecting a lack of genuine Jewish literacy.[22] This is not to deny the real privileges gained over time, including statehood, but to situate them within a context of complexity and ongoing struggle. It is particularly harmful when individuals who are disconnected from their Jewish heritage or who identify only with defensive or reactive aspects of Jewish experience, assume the authority to define what it means to be Jewish for others. Such positions are often informed by a disorganized attachment to their own Jewish identity, resulting in perspectives that are partial, defensive, and limited, and that fail to account for the rich, complex, and historically continuous nature of Jewish identity as an ethno-religious civilization.

Psychic health and intersubjectivity, which are the pinnacle of social connectedness, require the capacity for integration, relationality, and flexibility. A secure attachment entails being oneself, among other selves, while offering recognition and dignity both to oneself and to others. This pluralistic model has been increasingly replaced by hierarchical thinking amid the ideological polarization dominating modern American collective life. Comparative suffering has come to replace collective understanding. Santoro et al. (2025) note that shame is shaped by early relational experiences and functions as a regulatory mechanism for social belonging. Appeals to shame carry heightened power and primal force for those with double consciousness, as the tension between conflicting identities amplifies their vulnerability to internalized social judgments and deepens the experience of psychic fragmentation.

To explore how these dynamics play out in mental health practice, I spoke with Malka Shaw, a clinician who integrates Jewish literacy into her work, particularly in helping groups and communities understand, identify, and address instances of internalized anti-Jewish bias. Her interventions target the field in which antisemitism grows and spreads, working communally to undo some of its powerful and negating effects. As Pogue-White (2002) emphasizes, courageous dialogue is a crucial first step toward both personal and collective transformation. This chapter seeks to take that step. And while the following case study examines one approach toward addressing a particular internalized bias, the findings have broader applicability.

Psychoeducation, Self-Reclamation, and Cultural Humility

Malka Shaw, LCSW, is a trauma therapist in private practice and founder of Kesher Shalom Projects, an initiative she launched to address the psychological impact of antisemitism within the Jewish community and beyond by promoting cultural competency, resilience-building, and community support. Although Shaw's training is rooted in cognitive behavioral therapy and trauma theory, and my own in psychoanalysis, I recognized that her trauma-informed and communal workshop approach aligns significantly with psychoanalytic understandings of social and collective intervention. I met with Shaw on two occasions to explore the theoretical and practical applications of her organization and to further contextualize her work within my broader inquiry into internalized antisemitism as a developmental and attachment-related wound. Her trauma-informed, community-centered approach offers valuable insights into how collective and individual trauma intersect, deepening our understanding of the psychological processes through which internalized antisemitism is maintained and potentially transformed.

As a trauma therapist and clinical social worker serving a diverse population, Malka Shaw assumed the role of communal educator following Hamas's October 7 massacre on Israel. Shaw witnessed how the event reawakened historical trauma embedded in the collective psyche. The meaning of October 7 is deeply shaped by one's sociocultural position as both subject and object within larger social narratives. Through the American Jewish lens, the event stirred powerful defenses within the Jewish diaspora. Cosgrove (2024) writes, "[T]he pogrom-like nature of the day was intended as and understood to be an attack not just on Israel, but on global Jewry" (p. xxi). In response, Shaw witnessed and described a mobilization of psychological mechanisms rooted in resilience, protection, defense, and collective identity being activated in response to this trauma and threat. Shaw noted how October 7 did not exist in isolation; rather, it stirred intergenerational wounds shaped by centuries of persecution, displacement, and existential threat, reigniting ancestral fears and survival anxieties that reside just beneath the surface of contemporary Jewish identity. Cosgrove (2024) writes,

> October 7th and its reverberations ... is best understood as an accelerant or catalyst— not something entirely new. All the fault lines—relations between Israel and diaspora Jewry, antisemitism, the double consciousness of American Jews—have long been with us. October 7th brought them into full relief and gave them new urgency.
>
> (p. xxiii)

At the same time, this event emphasized a very different meaning to those outside the American Jewish diaspora[23] experience, one that includes the ongoing trauma of dispossession experienced by Palestinians from the establishment of Israel as a country in 1948 (the *Nakba*). This perspective resonated most with many Americans, especially in the wake of the cultural shift toward anti-racism sparked by the global rise of the Black Lives Matter movement, offering a framework that felt accessible as compared to the *less intelligible* understanding of Jewish intergenerational trauma and the complex presentations it takes.[24] From this perspective, October 7 symbolized an eruption of long-suppressed rage and grief rooted in statelessness, occupation, and systemic marginalization, which provided a psychological rationalization for the extremist violence and the erasure and minimization of Jewish pain and suffering as a result of the attack. Philosophers such as Franz Fanon and Judith Butler were invoked by many to explain away the brutality of the day, framing it as a proportionate response to the suffering of statelessness and systemic prejudice experienced by Palestinians at the hands of the Israeli state. While these frameworks contextualize violence as protest within histories of oppression, their application in this instance risked collapsing moral and political complexity, reducing unspeakable brutality to a symbolic act, and in doing so, foreclosed the possibility of mutual recognition or grief. Such interpretations may offer intellectual coherence but ultimately fail to contend with the psychological reality of trauma and the ethical imperative to hold violence accountable, regardless of its origin.

Although the attack has been interpreted by some as a challenge to expressions of Jewish power and the political marginalization of Palestinian identities by the State of Israel, it *definitively* foreclosed any possibility for intersubjective relationality. Israel's subsequent response of war foreclosed the possibility of intersubjective relationality further, as we know the context of war activates primitive defenses that undermine relational thinking in all subjects (Bion, 1961). The sheer brutality of the attacks and the responses they provoked, followed by the humanitarian crisis that ensued in the Gaza Strip, eliminated the conditions necessary for intersubjective recognition or relationality, not only in the Middle East but also here in America, both within the Jewish community and between the Jewish community and others. The internet and its algorithms have further entrenched individuals within silos of their own belief systems, thereby deepening divisions and eroding any possibility for genuine intersubjective engagement. The psychic meaning of the event is thus radically different depending on one's sociocultural location within this conflict, as well as one's internal psychological identifications to power and powerlessness, revealing layers of complexity, trauma, and insecure attachment. The difficulty of sustaining intersubjective space when collective narratives are shaped by mutual threat and historical grievance over a long time was plain for all to see (Volkan, 1997). The "field" here was ripe for intervention. Psychoanalytically, the challenge lies in holding space for multiple truths without collapsing into binary thinking, recognizing that trauma forecloses empathy and promotes either self-exceptionalism or self-erasure, and yet it is precisely empathy for the self and the Other that is needed to interrupt the cycles of dehumanization and retaliatory violence.

Shaw recognizes that the American Jewish community's post-trauma disorientation, grief, and identity fragmentation demand patient, collective repair, a process not only about reclaiming Jewish identity but also about securing the foundation for intersubjective connection itself. The absence of this secure attachment threatens both communal integrity and the very possibility of meaningful relationality. Following attacks that revived antisemitism to levels unseen since World War II,

Shaw developed workshops rooted in Jewish literacy, historical awareness, and psychoanalytic trauma theory to create a secure base amid widespread invalidation. These workshops move beyond information, inviting participants into deep self-inquiry and relational reflection. They explore how antisemitism functions externally in ideology, marginalization, and denial, as well as internally, as a destabilizing psychic force. Listening to her, I was reminded of Vogt's (2012) concept of perpetrator introjects, malevolent dissociative states that take root via introjection under conditions of extreme stress, in which survivors implicitly learn to mimic the beliefs and behaviors of an abuser. In this light, internalized antisemitism can be understood as an atmospheric foreign body that leaves a psychic imprint formed through repeated exposure to external hatred and cold indifference, one that becomes lodged within the self and disrupts both authentic connection and self-possession.

Through a combination of experiential dialogue, psychoeducation, and embodied practice, Shaw cultivates a space where participants can begin to reengage with their Jewish heritage as both a personal anchor and a political identity. Central to her work is what she calls the "BRIDGE" technique, a relational model designed to foster critical reflection without triggering defensiveness, thereby reclaiming self-autonomy from the corrosive effects of internalized antisemitism. Drawing from well-established psychological tools, Shaw adapts them toward a distinctly cultural aim: restoring a sense of security in one's identity. In her model, **B** stands for *boundaries*, **R** for *reflection*, **I** for *introducing cognitive dissonance*, **D** for *deconstructing emotional barriers to curiosity*, **G** for *generating alternatives in a co-regulated dyad that honors uniqueness and multiplicity*, and **E** for *empowering individuals to explore and define that multiplicity in creative, affirming ways*.

Shaw's approach rests on the psychoanalytic premise that identity formed under chronic or intermittent conditions of invalidation often becomes structured around defensive postures. While these defenses may serve a protective function, they can also obscure self-knowledge and inhibit meaningful intersubjective engagement, a dynamic that can be observed across other marginalized identities as well. For example, incorporating pride may function as affirmation of identity in the face of historical oppression for any number of marginalized peoples. The pride though is not rooted in an essentialist notion of what it means to be Jewish, Black, Queer, etc. Instead, hyphenated identities hold space for plurality, contradiction, and self-definition, allowing for a more expansive and evolving sense of belonging. As Brittney Cooper (2018) articulates in her nuanced exploration of Black-American female subjectivity, identity is not a fixed essentialist truth but rather a space of becoming, shaped by history, struggle, and imagination. Seen through this light, Shaw's work, then, is not merely pedagogical but reparative, a communal intervention aimed at loosening the internalized constraints of antisemitism in order to make room for new modes of meaning-making, mutual recognition, and collective self-resilience.

In these workshops, Malka Shaw illuminates how the polarized and Jewish illiterate ideological landscape of contemporary times fractures Jewish-identified people and their allies, leaving them vulnerable to a painful process of identity diffusion and collapse. This dynamic unfolds on the already unstable foundation of American Jewish identity, as Cosgrove explains. In sociopolitical terms, "the bargain of emancipation" for American Jews required that, "in return for becoming fully integrated citizens, [American] Jews were expected (or expected themselves) to shed their distinctive religious and cultural markers and adopt secular lifestyles" (Cosgrove, 2024, p. 37). Already lacking in a capacity to stand in the spaces of multiple identifications well enough, the trauma of October 7 further undermined a space for self-possession to develop. Shaw shares, "Hate doesn't just attack ideas; it fractures who we are to ourselves." By exploring the collective impact of macro-traumatic invalidation on Jewish individuals' capacity for self-determination and self-definition, she frames internalized antisemitism not simply as a personal struggle but as a groupthink phenomenon. Fractured identity leaves one vulnerable to internalizing false narratives, which can deepen insecure attachment by making it difficult to reconcile external hostility with one's internal sense of self. The collective experience of anti- Jewish bias further undermines autonomy, leaving Jewish individuals trapped in a web that erodes their capacity to self-define and self-determine.

In one of her workshops, it became strikingly clear how traumatic collective Jewish experience is systematically denied by both non-Jews and insecurely attached Jews alike, even as other marginalized experiences are increasingly witnessed and centered. This denial is not simply an alternate interpretation of events, but it is a form of epistemic violence, one that deliberately obscures the scale and reality of Jewish dehumanization.[25] Through rhetorical strategies that minimize, distort, or erase Jewish pain, these narratives flatten identity and delegitimize the complexity of Jewish historical and psychological life. Importantly, Jews are not immune to reproducing this kind of epistemological violence, especially toward those with whom there has been long-term conflict. However, the actions of some Israeli Jewish leaders do not define Jewish identity, just as the actions of Hamas do not define Palestinian identity, even though both can and do perpetuate harm. What's essential to name here is that Jewish identity is increasingly asked to exist only through disavowal, to be intelligible only when it conforms to dominant moral frameworks that cast Jewish power as inherently suspect. Jessica Benjamin's concept of the "doer–done-to" relational field helps make sense of this. In such a dynamic, subjects are locked into binary roles: either empowered agent or powerless victim. Jewish identity is thus reduced to a caricature, either a symbol of privileged invulnerability or historical victimhood without contemporary legitimacy. This dynamic invalidates Jewish trauma and reinforces antisemitic tropes that associate Jewishness with unearned power. The denial becomes not just interpersonal but structural: a strategy to maintain dominant narratives through what Shaw describes as moral disengagement, or the internal suspension of ethical standards used to justify harm.

This phenomenon appeared as a recurrent theme encountered among mental health professionals in workshops, who shared the kinds of statements they regularly heard from colleagues:

- *Come on, that's not antisemitic.*
- *I'm just antizionist, not antisemitic.*
- *You're being too sensitive.*
- *Jews aren't a credible source on antisemitism—they're too emotional.*

Such statements leave Jewish Americans whose attachment remains insecure extremely vulnerable to self-alienation, self-hatred and hatred of the Other. This is the defining wound of disorganized attachment: the impossibility of being held in one's wholeness.

Moral disengagement or traumatic invalidation in this context functions like the defense structure of an abusive or emotionally unavailable caregiver (Bar-Halpern & Wolfman, 2025). The message is: *You're too much. Too sensitive. Not credible when you speak of your pain.* The result is a profound breakdown in trust, where the subject is caught in a perpetual impasse, seeking connection from systems that repeatedly mirror back threat or indifference. One never knows which "version" of the system (caregiver) they will encounter. This unreliable mirroring erodes self-trust and distorts moral clarity. It confuses the inner moral compass, a key injury in disorganized attachment. It also gives rise to a kind of disorganized superego, where therapeutic ideals are not experienced as care but as surveillance. *You must accept my reality, but your reality is wrong. You must tolerate discomfort but not speak of it. You must reframe your pain, but only in ways that protect the social order of which you long to belong.*

When Jewish subjects are asked to split between cultural identity and political credibility, between ancestral grief and contemporary acceptability, the result is an incoherent internal map of belonging. They become, simultaneously, hyper-visible and erased, over-identified and disbelieved.[26] It is a psychic double bind, one that is not just ideological but affective and bodily. It shows up as shame, vigilance, dissociation, and the repeated reenactment of abandonment within institutions that claim to offer care. This is the inner cost of being rendered unintelligible. And yet, naming it—bringing this disorganization into awareness—is the first act of repair.

Case Example

In a training for mental health professionals, Shaw offered a clinical example that illustrates the application of the BRIDGE technique with a young Jewish American college student just beginning her first semester of school after the events of October 7. The student shared that she was sharing a dorm room with another student who identified as pro-Palestinian and expressed support for Hamas's efforts to reclaim land for the Palestinian people. This dynamic activated a painful internal split for the Jewish student: to honor her connection to her Jewish identity risked social ostracization, while to belong socially at school seemed to require self-erasure.

Initially, the student attempted to clarify her position, that her Jewishness and support for the existence of a Jewish state did not preclude her also supporting Palestinian sovereignty and rejecting the actions of the Israeli government that went against this. But her roommate was unable to hold the intersubjective space required to allow for such nuance. Her roommate interpreted her Jewish self-identification and refusal to denounce Zionism as inherently dehumanizing to Palestinians. The relational field became one in which the young woman felt enormous pressure to internalize self-hatred in order to belong.

Shaw guided the student through the BRIDGE model in sequential steps. The first step, boundaries, involved creating an embodied sense of physical and psychological safety through bilateral stimulation, guided eye movements, a core component of EMDR, that have been effectively used to calm the nervous system and prepare individuals for trauma processing. Shaw emphasized that without a space in which one can simply *be*, the nervous system remains in a reactive state. She helped the student carve out a boundary within the shared dorm room, a space that was not for debate, defense, or ideological engagement but simply for presence. Importantly, the bilateral stimulation shifted the exercise from a purely cognitive task to a bottom-up, somatically integrated experience. As Shaw noted, no one imagines their way into secure attachment, it must be felt. Soma safety precedes conceptual integration.

Only once that secure space was established and consistently available could the work of reflection begin. From this grounded position, the student could begin to explore how current political and social events, both domestic and abroad, were impacting her sense of Jewish identity. With time and containment, she could notice the defenses that arose, including moments of self-blame, and become curious about them. *What aspects of herself did she feel she had to relinquish in order to belong? What parts could remain intact? How could she hold the pain of others without surrendering her own integrity? Could she resist the pull of ideological conformity while still remaining open to perspectives that were not her own*? Crucially, Shaw emphasized that such reflection was not possible in the absence of felt safety.

The next stage introduced cognitive dissonance, where Shaw gently supported the student in tolerating complexity. For example, they explored the incongruity between the roommate's stated values of justice and inclusion and her participation in acts like tearing down posters of kidnapped Israelis, seeing Jewish pain as "propaganda." Could the liberation of one group be achieved through the erasure of another? Similarly, the student was invited to explore her own limitations: was she less able to empathize with Palestinian Americans when she felt personally threatened or unseen?

This opened the door to deconstructing emotional barriers to curiosity. Having recognized that self-erasure was not aligned with her values of diversity and pluralism, the student could begin to reclaim her capacity for curiosity. Shaw helped her notice who in her environment could tolerate and hold the complexity of the moment and to seek out those connections. Understanding the developmental importance of peer relationships at this stage of life was key. Peer validation, or lack thereof, had the power to facilitate or block meaningful engagement.

Next, they moved to generating alternatives for managing conflict that could not be resolved. The student learned to establish boundaries with her roommate, clarifying when, how, and if she could engage in conversation and when she could not. She invited her roommate to do the same. This mutual regard allowed for the emergence of new relational configurations. While they did not influence one another's political positions, they were able to coexist with mutual respect.

Finally, in the empowering to explore and define phase, the work continued as the student grappled with how to inhabit her Jewish identity with pride in an environment where it was widely misunderstood and often appropriated or politicized by those who did not share it. She continued to wrestle with what it means to be Jewish in a space where nuance is often flattened and identity reduced to symbol.

Introducing this technique experientially to participants facilitated the internalization of greater security in their Jewish identity, not through foreclosure or retreat into rigidity, but by expanding their capacity for intersubjective engagement across difference. In this way, the intervention worked at the level of both structure and symbol, supporting the movement from defensive postures organized around grievance and persecutory identification toward a more integrated and developmentally mature sense of self. Here, identity is not organized through trauma alone, but through the capacity to tolerate complexity, mourn loss, and remain open to the other without abandoning the self.

Conclusion: Promoting Secure Connections in Collective Spaces

Identity destabilization undermines an individual's ability to develop a flexible and coherent sense of self, which is essential for engaging in meaningful intersubjective relationality. Whether the Other or the self becomes objectified poses a risk to intersubjective connection. The capacity to relate to others in a way that acknowledges mutual subjectivity, difference, and authentic connection requires self-knowledge and self-possession. When a person's sense of identity is persistently fragmented or eroded by the biases of the host or dominant culture, it disrupts their ability to trust both themselves and others, creating barriers to forming deep, reciprocal relationships. Shaw educates participants on the wide-ranging neurological effects of chronic destabilization, including cognitive rigidity, diminished critical thinking, reduced empathy, increased conformity, polarized thinking, fear-based decision-making, mistrust, learned helplessness, resistance to change, and the suppression of individual autonomy. The rigid adherence to external narratives is best understood then as an attempt to protect themselves from further confusion or pain. While these defenses may offer temporary relief, they ultimately hinder vulnerability and openness, which are critical for genuine intersubjective engagement. These effects may be felt by all marginalized identities who hold an insecure attachment.

As a result, the possibility of achieving authentic relational connection becomes increasingly elusive. Cosgrove (2024) writes, "To live a hyphenated life is not an outcome or a destination, it is a perpetual state of being. It means that life is a balancing act between the competing commitments within each of us" (p. 3). Without a stable foundation of selfhood, a marginalized individual will struggle to participate fully in shared understanding and mutual recognition, remaining caught in a cycle of isolation and disconnection. Recognition must be mutual to be felt. It begins internally. With one part of self-seeing another part of self through meta-dialogue[27] (Dobrich, 2020).

Shaw is not suggesting that the Jewish narrative is supreme or singular, but rather that it belongs within a multicultural mosaic—alongside other groups—where it is commonly understood that marginalized peoples have the right to self-define how they carry their heritage and their responsibilities to one another, and to the cultures around them.

When an individual's sense of self becomes dependent on defining or delimiting the identity of another, the relational field shifts from one of intersubjectivity to one of control and domination. From a psychoanalytic and trauma-informed perspective, this dynamic often reflects unresolved trauma or narcissistic injury, in which the self seeks coherence not through internal integration, but through the external *regulation* of others. Rather than recognizing the Other as a separate subject with their own complex interiority, the Other becomes a projection screen used to stabilize a fragmented or threatened sense of self. This forecloses the possibility of mutual recognition, a cornerstone of intersubjective relating, and instead reenacts patterns of relational trauma, where power and control are substituted for empathy and attunement.

Working through internalized antisemitism ultimately means acquiring a secure attachment as *both* a Jew and an American. It is, in the words of Rabbi Cosgrove (2024), "A vision whereby the Jewish people, and all people, can live peaceably together, amid their differences. A vision of tribalism without triumphalism, affiliation without parochialism, peoplehood without ethnocentrism" (p. 13). And psychoanalytically speaking, no one can have relational recognition without being granted the capacity to recognize oneself. Though this particular example focused on the Jewish American experience in a post-October 7 climate, this model of working through internalized bias due to one's marginalized cultural position as a subject is applicable to all peoples who share a "hyphenated" existence. Malka Shaw is but one example of an educator clinician utilizing applied psychoanalysis toward social repair.

Understanding bias as a legacy of insecure attachment invites us to move beyond the intrapsychic realm of the individual patient and the traditional one-to-one analytic setting. It calls for engagement within communal and intersubjective spaces where the dynamics of cultural identity and self-sovereignty are negotiated and reworked. From a psychoanalytic perspective, internalized bias is not merely a personal pathology or adaptation but a manifestation of unconscious identifications and defenses shaped by historical trauma and relational disruptions *across* generations. These unconscious processes are embedded in the social field and transmitted within communities, impacting collective subjectivity and the possibility for intersubjective authentic relationality profoundly. Addressing internalized bias therefore requires engaging with these broader relational matrices, creating a reparative encounter that can contain ambivalence, redistribute narrative authority, acknowledge disavowed aspects of identity, and support new symbolic integrations. This shift allows psychoanalytic work to extend its reach, supporting not only individual psychic restructuring but also communal healing, intercultural relations, and cultural transformation.

Acknowledgments

I extend my sincere gratitude to Sheldon Itzkowitz, Sarah Milburn, Irit Felsen, Yael Shy, Yamille Mason, and Anna Mitchell for their insightful and generous feedback on earlier drafts of this chapter. Their meaningful contributions and critical perspectives greatly enriched the development of this work. I'd also like to thank Malka Shaw for generously agreeing to be interviewed and for sharing her work with me, which provided invaluable insights that informed this chapter.

Notes

1 By "dominant," I do not mean superior or positive but rather those groups that hold normative power: the authority to shape material, psychological, and social conditions within a given society (Foucault, 1980).

2 Benjamin (1988) defines recognition as a mutual *and* intersubjective process where both self and Other acknowledge each other's subjectivity and autonomy. It involves being able to see the Other not as an object but as a separate, autonomous subject with their own feelings, desires, and history.

3 Pluralism views relational life as a dynamic process where various groups (e.g., economic, social, cultural, and political organizations) compete and collaborate to shape policies and represent different interests within society (Dahl, 1961). Jessica Benjamin, Stephen Frosh, Donald Meltzer, Thomas Ogden, Paul Wachtel, Irving Yalom, and Lew Aron are key psychoanalytic thinkers who have explored pluralism within psychoanalysis whether explicitly or implicitly, emphasizing the multiplicity of subjectivities, perspectives, and interpretations within the mind, therapeutic dyad, schools of thought, and society writ large.

4 J. M. Berger (2018) studies extremism and reveals that extremism is not simply about holding radical views but about how those views position others as existential threats, thereby justifying hostility, violence, or uncaring indifference.

5 Faimberg uses this term to refer to a collapse or compression of generational boundaries, where the unconscious conflicts, desires, and actual traumas of previous generations are not properly symbolized, and go on to invade the psychic space of the next generation, as if the generations are "telescoped" into one another.
6 Contreras (2023) describes intergenerational trauma related to identity as *Aggregated Traumatization Syndrome*, a layering of inherited alterations, insecure attachments, systemic adversity, and the individualized traumatizing agents experienced within a single life (p. 277).
7 Dave Chappelle, Jerry Seinfeld, Ali Wong, and Hannah Gadsby exemplify performers who critically engage with and deconstruct cultural archetypes linked to various marginalized identities.
8 Contemporary community psychoanalysis stands on the foundational contributions of theorists such as Karen Horney, Harry Stack Sullivan, and William Alanson White, who critically challenged early psychoanalysis's exclusive intrapsychic focus by foregrounding the social, relational, and cultural determinants of the psyche.
9 Epstein (2018) uses the term "scaregiver" to refer to an attachment figure who functions as a source of fear rather than safety, in the context of trauma. Rather than providing comfort, protection, and secure base support, a "scaregiver" is experienced as frightening, unpredictable, or threatening, contributing to disorganized attachment, fragmentation of self, and defensive adaptations in the developing psyche.
10 One could argue that attachment dynamics also exist between individuals and their marginalized communities, through which *many* forms of cultural resilience are transmitted, though this realm is not the focus of this chapter. Instead, the emphasis here is on how internalized bias arises primarily from the dynamics of the ingroup–outgroup relationship, particularly in response to the dominant culture's projections, exclusions, and failures of recognition.
11 Freud (1931) and Fromm (1956) both emphasized belonging as a psychological and social necessity. Freud via the dynamics of group identification and mourning, and Fromm through the foundational human needs of rootedness and relatedness. While Freud's work illuminates how we forge belonging through identification with group ideals, Fromm shows us that authentic belonging must arise from internal integration, such as creative love, purposeful connection, and reconciliation of freedom with communion.
12 For example, Eng and Han (2019) describe racial dissociation as encompassing racial melancholia, a collective, historically grounded psychic condition in which racialized losses and unfulfilled social expectations shape subjectivity across generations among Asian Americans.
13 A likely critique of this chapter is the choice to illustrate ethnocultural identity and attachment with a Jewish case example rather than a racialized example in which "passing" is not possible. My intention in selecting a

Jewish case is to highlight the complexity of minority identity in the United States, where marginalization is not always linked to visible markers, and where the capacity to "pass" can obscure the psychological and relational burdens carried by those who occupy ambiguous or contested minority positions. Jewish identity, racially diverse, historically persecuted, and yet frequently misperceived as fully assimilated, illuminates a distinct dimension of ethnocultural attachment: the chronic negotiation between visibility and invisibility. The ability to be mistaken for part of the dominant culture does not remove inherited trauma, sociocultural vulnerability, or internalized pressure to minimize or conceal one's difference. In fact, it can intensify identity conflict, contributing to attachment disorganization, in which the self must navigate contradictory demands of belonging and self-protection, safety and erasure. By using a Jewish case example, I aim to broaden the conversation and highlight that ethnocultural identity and its psychological dimensions can take many forms, not all of which are tied to visible racial markers. This example demonstrates how minority stress, internalized narratives, and oscillation between threat and conditional acceptance can produce disorganization in the attachment system, situating Jewish experience within the wider American landscape of race, ethnicity, culture, and relational development.

14 Erlich (2025) writes,

> It is true that antisemitism may be invoked defensively, yet I maintain that this can also be a false allegation, designed to ignore and deny antisemitism where it exists.... Antisemitism is an amazingly unique phenomenon, transcending generational and geographical boundaries, nor is it something of the past.
> (p. 168)

Throughout this discussion, I use the terms *antisemitism* and *anti-Jewish bias* interchangeably. However, given the politicization of the term *antisemitism*, I find *anti-Jewish bias* to be a more direct and accessible formulation.

15 Sandmeyer (2024) illustrates the frequent misattribution of "privilege" to Jewishness, showing how stereotypes can be unconsciously absorbed even in work that seeks to acknowledge the complexities of American Jewish identity. The paper characterizes historically developed resilient capacities exclusively as unearned racial "privilege," though these capacities are neither the product of favoritism nor unearned advantage and always exist alongside ongoing experiences of significant Othering.

16 There is no shortage of examples illustrating this double bind in Jewish history. One striking instance is the early Reform movement in Germany, which shifted Shabbat observance from Saturday to Sunday, despite Shabbat having been observed from Friday sundown since ancient times. This change reflected not just assimilation but a culturally disorganized attachment, signaling the tension between preservation and belonging (Meyer, 1988). An example within Sephardic Jewish culture is "Conversos":

Jews in Spain and Portugal who were forcibly converted to Christianity during the late Middle Ages but secretly maintained Jewish rituals and practices in private (Perry, 1991). A more contemporary example of this cultural double bind appears in queer Jewish communities, where individuals have been asked not to wear visibly identifiable Jewish markers at Pride marches and/or to denounce their "Zionism." These restrictions, often justified as efforts to avoid "nationalistic" imagery, not only sideline Jewish visibility within queer spaces but also conflate individual Jewish identity with the actions of the Israeli state, collapsing a rich diasporic identity into a singular political narrative (A Wider Bridge, 2025).

17 Of course, some individuals maintain a secure attachment to both their Jewish identity and the non-Jewish world; there are securely attached Jews. While it would be valuable to examine the conditions that support this integration, space constraints prevent a detailed discussion in this chapter.

18 There are numerous examples, but a significant one involves moneylending. In the Middle Ages, Christian prohibitions against usury barred Christians from lending money with interest, leading Jews to assume this role. This dynamic is exemplified by the figure of Shylock in *The Merchant of Venice*, who personifies antisemitic resentment toward Jewish moneylenders, a stereotype that persists to this day (Horn, 2021; Kamen, 1998).

19 Freeman (2021) observes that contemporary identity politics frequently relies on a rigid binary positioning subjects as either "White oppressors" or "people of color" as the oppressed. Within this framework, Jews are often misrecognized as members of the dominant "White" class and are thus denied access to the social capital of marginalization that underpins allyship. This misrecognition not only obscures the historical trauma and ongoing vulnerability of Jewish identity but also effaces the psychic reality of antisemitism itself. The consequence, Freeman argues, is a structural exclusion of Jews from progressive coalitions, where solidarity is unevenly allocated and Jewish suffering is rendered imperceptible.

20 Roisman et al. (2002) define earned-secure attachment as the process through which individuals who experienced early attachment insecurity develop a coherent and secure attachment representation in adulthood, facilitated by subsequent reparative relationships.

21 For example, Griffin et al. (2020) provide a critical analysis of racialized dynamics in psychoanalytic training, highlighting anti-Black racism, classism, and xenophobia. Yet their paper largely leaves anti-Jewish bias and antisemitism unacknowledged and, at times, enacted—reflecting the very institutional patterns they critique in relation to other groups. One illustration is the title *The Secret Society*, which echoes the stereotype of Jews secretly controlling institutions.

22 Expressions of Jewish power carried out by the Jewish state are not equivalent to collective Jewish identity itself. Just as the actions of any diaspora's

homeland government do not define the culture or identity of its people, the political actions of Israel should not be taken as representative of all Jewish individuals or their collective identity.

23 It is important to note that not all American Jews identified with the particular Jewish American experience described here. As noted earlier in the chapter, the nature of one's attachment relationship to both one's Jewish identity and the host culture significantly shapes the psychological response. Additionally, there has never been a monolithic category of Jewish experience. For those with a more tenuous connection to their Jewish identity and a stronger affiliation with the dominant culture, the response to October 7 may have more closely resembled that of their non-Jewish American counterparts, filtered less through communal trauma/resiliency and more through progressive American political frameworks. In practice, this is often the only Jewish perspective represented in mainstream spaces, including many psychoanalytic journals, because it aligns with the dominant progressive cultural imperative to center those perceived as underserved or marginalized, which in this case does not include the Jews. This bias in framing inadvertently obscures the diversity of Jewish experience and forecloses more complex or ambivalent expressions of Jewish identity, grief, and vulnerability while reinforcing antisemitic tropes.

24 A study of *The New York Times* coverage between October 2023 and mid-2024 found a disproportionate expression of empathy toward Palestinians: 46% of articles expressed empathy *only* toward Palestinians, while just 10.5% did so for Israelis. Headlines similarly favored the Palestinian perspective in 55% of top news headlines versus only 5.8% favoring Israeli narratives. Of course, the study also reveals the binary nature of the conflict (Sigan, 2024).

25 For example, Bendov (2025) notes, "Most clinicians have not been trained to identify signs and symptoms directly related to antisemitism, have limited understanding of antisemitism, including its definition and history, and lack competency models in the literature to guide their practice" (p. 1).

26 See Judith Herman, *Truth and Repair: How Trauma Survivors Envision Justice* (2023), in which she describes how survivors are often simultaneously erased and disbelieved by both institutions and communities. Herman emphasizes that this dual negation produces profound psychic and bodily effects and that acknowledgment and bearing witness are essential first steps toward repair. The dynamics she describes for trauma survivors closely parallel the double bind experienced by Jewish subjects negotiating between cultural identity, political credibility, and ancestral grief.

27 I define meta-dialogue as the intrapsychic conversation among fractured parts of the self: an internal process that seeks to move beyond enacted or dissociated behavior toward reflective communication, ultimately facilitating mourning and relational integration.

References

A Wider Bridge. (2025, June). Unsafe spaces: Addressing antisemitism against LGBTQ+ Jews and ensuring pride safety. https://awiderbridge.org/wp-content/uploads/Unsafe-Spaces-A-Wider-Bridge-Report-2025.pdf

Apprey, M. (2023). *Transgenerational haunting in psychoanalysis: Toxic errands* (W.F.Cornell,Ed.; 1sted.). Routledge. https://doi.org/10.4324/9781003389026

Bar-Halpern, M., & Wolfman, J. (2025). Traumatic invalidation in the Jewish community after October 7. *Journal of Human Behavior in the Social Environment, 35*(8), 1366–1393. https://doi.org/10.1080/10911359.2025.2503441

Bendov, A. (2025). Addressing antisemitism in psychotherapy: A trauma-informed and culturally responsive approach, *Journal of Human Behavior in the Social Environment, 35*(8), 1467–1476. https://doi.org/10.1080/10911359.2025.2545536

Benjamin, J. (1988). *The bonds of love: Psychoanalysis, feminism, and the problem of domination*. Pantheon Books.

Benjamin, J. (1995). *Like subjects, love objects: Essays on recognition and sexual difference*. Yale University Press.

Berger, J. M. (2018). *Extremism*. MIT Press.

Berry, J. W. (1997). Immigration, acculturation, and adaptation. *Applied Psychology. An International Review, 46*(1), 5–34. https://doi.org/10.1111/j.1464-0597.1997.tb01087.x

Bion, W. R. (1961). *Experiences in groups*. Tavistock Publications.

Contreras, A. (2023). *Traumatization and its aftermath: A systemic approach to understanding and treating trauma disorders*. Routledge.

Cooper, B. (2018). *Eloquent rage: A Black feminist discovers her superpower*. St. Martin's Press.

Cosgrove, E. J. (2024). *For such a time as this: On being Jewish today*. Harvest.

Dahl, R. A. (1961). *Who governs? Democracy and power in an American city*. Yale University Press.

Dobrich, J. (2020). An elegy for motherless daughters: Dissociation, multiplicity, and mourning. *Psychoanalytic Perspectives, 17*(3), 366–384.

Du Bois, W. E. B. (1903). *The souls of Black folk*. A. C. McClurg & Co.

Echegoyen, R. (2022, Winter). Abandoning the analytic frame: Psychoanalysis and racism. *Division Review*.

Ellenberger, H. F. (1970). *The discovery of the unconscious: The history and evolution of dynamic psychiatry*. Basic Books.

Eng, D. L., & Han, S. (2019). *Racial melancholia, racial dissociation: On the social and psychic lives of Asian Americans*. Duke University Press.

Epstein, O. B. (2018). From proximity seeking to relationship seeking: Working towards separation from the "scaregivers." *Frontiers in the Psychotherapy of Trauma and Dissociation*, 2(1), 290–306.

Erlich, S. (2025). Is psychoanalysis relevant to the Israeli–Palestinian conflict? *The International Journal of Psychoanalysis, 106*(1), 165–173. https://doi.org/10.1080/00207578.2025.2453295

Faimberg, H. (1988). The telescoping of generations: Genealogy of certain identifications. *Contemporary Psychoanalysis*, *24*(1), 99–118. https://doi.org/10.1080/00107530.1988.10746222

Fanon, F. (2008). *Black skin, white masks* (C. L. Markmann, Trans.). Grove Press. (Original work published 1952).

Felsen, I. (2017). Adult-onset trauma and intergenerational transmission: Integrating empirical data and psychoanalytic theory. *Psychoanalysis, Self and Context*, *12*(1), 60–77.

Felsen, I. (2021). *Intergenerational trauma and cultural healing: A conversation that must continue*. Museum of Jewish Heritage.

Fonagy, P., Gergely, G., Jurist, E. L., & Target, M. (2002). *Affect regulation, mentalization, and the development of the self*. Other Press.

Foucault, M. (1980). *Power/knowledge: Selected interviews and other writings, 1972–1977* (C. Gordon, Ed.). Pantheon Books.

Freeman, B. M. (2021). *Jewish pride: Rebuilding a people*. Whitefox Publishing.

Freud, S. (1931). *Group psychology and the analysis of the ego* (J. Strachey, Trans.). Hogarth Press.

Fromm, E. (1956). *The art of loving*. Harper & Row.

Frosh, S. (2005). Jung and the Nazis: Some implications for psychoanalysis. *Psychoanalysis and History*, *7*(2), 253–271.

Gilman, S. L. (1985). *Difference and pathology: Stereotypes of sexuality, race, and madness*. Cornell University Press.

Griffin, C. D., Echegoyen, R., & Hyman, J. (2020). The secret society: Perspectives from a multiracial cohort. *Contemporary Psychoanalysis*, *56*(2–3), 282–304. https://doi.org/10.1080/00107530.2020.1777520

Harris, A. (2009). Gender as soft assembly. *Psychoanalytic Dialogues*, *19*(5), 513–528.

Hart, A. (2017). From multicultural competence to radical openness: A psychoanalytic engagement of otherness. *The American Psychoanalyst*, *51*(1), 17–20.

Herman, J. L. (2023). *Truth and repair: How trauma survivors envision justice*. Basic Books.

Horn, D. (2021). *People love dead Jews: Reports from a haunted present* (1st ed.). W. W. Norton & Company.

Kamen, H. (1998). *The Spanish Inquisition: A historical revision*. Yale University Press.

Kim, C. J. (1999). The racial triangulation of Asian Americans. *Politics & Society*, *27*(1), 105–138. https://doi.org/10.1177/0032329299027001005

Laub, D. (1992). Bearing witness, or the vicissitudes of listening. In S. Felman & D. Laub (Eds.), *Testimony: Crises of witnessing in literature, psychoanalysis, and history* (pp. 57–74). Routledge.

Meyer, M. A. (1988). *Response to modernity: A history of the reform movement in Judaism*. Wayne State University Press.

Mitchell, S. A. (2000). *Relationality: From attachment to intersubjectivity*. Analytic Press.

Perry, M. (1991). *The Jews and the Spanish Inquisition*. Jewish Publication Society.

Pogue-White, K. (2002). Surviving hating and being hated: Some personal thoughts about racism from a psychoanalytic perspective. *Contemporary Psychoanalysis*, *38*(3), 401–422. https://doi.org/10.1080/00107530.2002.10747173

Roisman, G. I., Padron, E., Sroufe, L. A., & Egeland, B. (2002). Earned-secure attachment status in retrospect and in prospect. *Child Development*, *73*(4), 1204–1219. https://doi.org/10.1111/1467-8624.00467

Sandmeyer, J. H. (2024). Transgenerational transmission of privilege and trauma: Locating Jewish experience in racial reckoning within psychoanalysis. *Contemporary Psychoanalysis*, *59*(3–4), 342–368. https://doi.org/10.1080/00107530.2024.2315007

Santoro, G., Sideli, L., Musetti, A., & Schimmenti, A. (2025). The relationship between childhood trauma and shame: The mediating role of dissociation. *European Journal of Investigation in Health, Psychology and Education*, *15*(8), 151. https://doi.org/10.3390/ejihpe15080151

Sigan, L. (2024, June 28). *Study reveals disturbing truth about the New York Times' coverage of the Gaza war. The Jewish Chronicle*.

Stephens, M. (2020). Getting next to ourselves: The interpersonal dimensions of double-consciousness. *Contemporary Psychoanalysis*, *56*(2–3), 201–225. https://doi.org/10.1080/00107530.2020.1776095

Stoute, B. J. (2019). Racial socialization and thwarted mentalization: Psychoanalytic reflections from the lived experience of James Baldwin's America. *The American Imago*, *76*(3), 335–357. https://doi.org/10.1353/aim.2019.0025

Vogt, R. (Ed.). (2012). *Perpetrator introjects: Psychotherapeutic diagnostics and treatment models*. Asanger Verlag.

Volkan, V. D. (1997). *Bloodlines: From ethnic pride to ethnic terrorism*. Farrar, Straus and Giroux.

Chapter 9

Knowing and Not Knowing About Our Climate Crisis

From Eco-Neglect to Mutual Sustenance on Planet Earth

Karen Hopenwasser

For each of us, small moments of awareness over decades yield the deep resonance of life on our home planet, Earth. With this awareness comes both great joy and enormous pain. I sit on the shore of a lake watching an eagle swoop down searching for prey. Yes, I know that this magnificent bird needs to eat. I recall the words of astronomer Carl Sagan, "the universe seems neither benign nor hostile, merely indifferent" (1980, p. 250).

As psychoanalysts and psychotherapists, we bear witness to so much suffering in this indifferent universe. Some of that suffering is caused by nature's indifference, in particular natural disasters. However, we live within an ecosystem uniquely shaped by human consciousness.

> Humans have evolved as a species with unique intellectual and cognitive capabilities to destroy the world in which they inhabit. This ability to destroy is a function of a loss of embodied wisdom, or a failure to integrate cognitive and embodied knowledge of complex systems. This reflects a Western ignorance and bias against Indigenous science and has contributed to profound social injustice.
>
> (Hopenwasser, 2024, p. 138)

Inaction about climate change is a failure to protect our children and can be considered a form of institutional child abuse.

The United Nations Committee on the Rights of the Child, in 2023, released general Comment 26, *On Children's Rights and the Environment with a Special Focus on Climate Change*, in which it "underscores that children have the right to a clean, healthy and sustainable environment."

DOI: 10.4324/9781003658382-10

An independent and international group of academics have proposed "that environmental degradation, including the climate crisis, is a form of structural violence against children" (Bourdillon et al., 2024, p. 1), defining structural violence as pertaining "to dominant institutions that impose systemic harms on a vulnerable group of individuals" (Bourdillon et al., 2024).

For so many years, I have borne witness to the impact of childhood abuse and neglect on individual patients. When I read Rebecca Solnit's "Call Climate Change What It Is: Violence," I was jolted into an awareness that smashed through the mental barrier between my consulting office and the outside world. Solnit states that "[c]limate change is global-scale violence, against places and species as well as against human beings" (2018, p. 86). If governments and corporations are considered to be institutions, then we need to recognize eco-neglect as institutional child abuse and child neglect.

How do we, as individual therapists, incorporate this awareness of inevitable future trauma into our everyday practice when we and our loved ones are directly threatened? Even though we are attentive to evidence of intergenerational transmission of trauma, appreciating the ways in which past trauma is transmitted down through generations (Apprey, 2023; Dobrich, 2026; Mucci, 2013, 2022; Salberg & Grand, 2016; Volkan, 2001, among many others), eco-neglect creates conditions that will inflict suffering right now as well as on future generations. If we do not notice this future threat, would that not be like sitting in a room in a burning building and saying, "Oh, the fire has not arrived in our room yet; let's continue with our business as usual"? As Donna Orange asked,

> Are we … so absorbed in our theories, and worse, in our theoretical and interdenominational disputes over who belongs and who does not, that we fail to notice that human-caused planetary warming threatens to destroy the world within which we practice our beloved profession?
>
> (2017, p. xii)

Fortunately, a growing number of individual therapists and therapist organizations (e.g., the Climate Psychology Alliance, Climate Psychiatry Alliance, the American Psychological Association Task Force on

Climate Change, the American Psychiatric Association Caucus on Climate Change) have taken on both advocacy and educational roles. Psychoanalyst Sally Weintrobe (2021), in her book *The Psychological Roots of the Climate Crisis: Neoliberal Exceptionalism and the Culture of Uncare* writes extensively about what she calls the culture of uncare, connecting political economy and human exceptionalism.

Some patients bring anxiety and concern about climate change into their psychotherapy sessions. When this happens, therapist and patient are knowingly working within the space of shared trauma (Saidipour, 2020; Tosone et al., 2012). But often anxieties about the future of our environment are unexpressed and the link between trauma and a rapidly changing planet remains unspoken. Just as in our work with adults mistreated as children, experiences of other chronic trauma and extreme stress are often dissociated.

I am going to draw some parallels between individual dissociative responses and larger social phenomena. Here is a simple clinical example of the complexity of dissociative adaptation. I have previously written about a patient, Ingrid, who came to me after many years of psychotherapy elsewhere to manage a binge eating disorder (Hopenwasser, 2016). Despite earnest effort in previous psychotherapies, she had not been able to control her binging and was at the start of our work morbidly obese. She described severe emotional abuse by a mother who lacked empathy and controlled her with cruel indifference to her suffering. She described her father as a funny and loving workaholic, who did not notice the cruelty of his wife to their children. He too struggled with obesity, and the two bonded together sneaking food at night. As an adult, she managed her suffering through workaholic achievement and dissociative binging.

Early in our therapy work, I used the words "abuse" and "cruelty" in a session. She appeared shocked. She knew that she felt mistreated, but she would never have described herself as abused. Putting into words what is known but also had been not known facilitated even more profound change in her life. Many years into our work, I recall so vividly, the session in which she sat forward in her chair, peering at me with intensity, and said, "They all knew, my teachers, my neighbors, friends of the family … why did no one say anything?"

While Ingrid is not "diagnosed" with a dissociative disorder, she clearly manifests dissociative moments when she both knows and not knows about her own traumatic experiences in childhood. She could masterfully manage complicated business deals, never forgetting a detail. Yet in her personal life, she often forgot facts about herself. A couple of years after treatment for an early and curable cancer, she would forget to tell new doctors that she had had cancer, and she would forget to go for follow-up checkups.

Ingrid was able to benefit from long-term therapy prior to our work together without ever being aware of her own experience of knowing and not knowing about her childhood trauma (Laub & Auerhahn, 1993). While I was grateful for the good treatment that she had before coming to me, the deepest, most satisfying changes occurred once we recognized the role of dissociation in her management of her suffering.

Currently, she still struggles with some bulimia. But she is no longer obese. She is no longer a workaholic. And she is more fully engaged in a community of friends. She is now able to talk with me about feelings of shame and has come to recognize her self-injurious rage that contributes to episodic binging.

It is more difficult to notice and understand a dissociative process in a larger system. This requires recognizing that dissociation can be normative and not necessarily in response to the stress of trauma. As Lisa Butler has stated, "[T]he primacy and ubiquity of dissociation in normal human experience are not well appreciated" (2006). Normative dissociation would include intense absorption in an activity such as playing music, sports, computer games, reading, and daydreaming. In addition, concepts of relationality are increasingly being applied to social and biological systems (Walsh et al., 2021; West et al., 2020; West et al., 2024). While recognizing the process of dissociation in individual mental organization is essential in the treatment of traumatized individuals, understanding the role of dissociation (as opposed to denial) on a larger social scale may also be essential to the survival of our species.

Professionals treating children began to formally recognize child abuse in the 19th and 20th centuries as children transitioned from being seen as the property of their fathers and as Western governments began to enact child labor laws (Committee on the Rights of the Child, 2023). The concept of the Battered Child Syndrome was first introduced in 1962 (Kempe et al., 1962). Article 3 of the United Nations Convention on the Rights of the Child, adopted in 1989 (though never ratified in the United States), articulates that the best interests of the child shall be primary. And now, in the 21st century, we have organizations such as Our Children's Trust, engaging in legal actions in the United States, and globally, to fight for the protection of our children's health (Our Children's Trust, n.d.).

Even though recognition of post-traumatic dissociation in our clinical work is steadily increasing, the concept of dissociation gets lost and found and then often lost again—historically from Janet in the 19th century, Freud before abandoning a trauma model, and Ferenczi mid-20th century, to more contemporary clinicians and theorists: Bromberg (1999), Howell and Itzkowitz (2016), Stern (2003), Chefetz (2015), and Dobrich (2021), among many others. There is an ever-growing literature addressing the diagnosis and treatment of trauma-induced dissociative adaptation. Can we take this knowledge to the level of group adaptation in an ecosystem? The phenomenon of human contributions to climate change may be one of the most flagrant examples of dissociated adaptation in an ecosystem.

One pathway to appreciating the self-similarity of large and small systems is simply listening and noticing. I treat individuals who have suffered abuse and neglect specifically perpetrated by other humans—organisms, unlike "the universe," capable of empathy. This work has stirred curiosity about the ways in which empathy manifests in moments of attunement. While our training teaches us to *think* about the unconscious mind, about transference and countertransference, about defense mechanisms, about projective identification, we do not necessarily learn to really listen. In her writings on *Radical Ethics*, Orange says, "It has become ever clearer, in theoretical worlds ranging from the classical through the Kleinian to the various intersubjectivities, that *how* the analyst listens determines, to a very great extent, *what* can be heard and responded to" (2020, p. 2).

Concepts of resonance, vibration, and rhythmic attunement are addressed less often in psychotherapy training (notable exceptions: somatic-based treatments, the writings of Bucci (2021), Knoblauch (2020), Trevarthen (1999–2000), and others who study maternal-infant rhythmic communication). When we somehow know things that have not been directly spoken, we call it uncanny communication, as if it is magical or paranormal to receive information that is not put into words. Somatic psychotherapies tend to focus on individual body experience such as the activation and collapse of the autonomic nervous system in response to chronic trauma, though Gendlin's concept of felt sense does recognize the deep resonance of information flow (Gendlin, 1981). We need to take this up a level, beyond the awareness of one's own body sensation. I have written elsewhere about the concept of a dissociative attunement in the therapeutic process (Hopenwasser, 2008, 2016). While this concept was born from intense clinical work with traumatized individuals who manifest a dissociative adaptation, it has emerged into a more generalized awareness of dissociated information not necessarily in response to individual traumas.

***

Back on the shoreline of the lake, I watch a flock of geese take flight. Within moments, they are flying in formation, perfectly communicating speed and direction for the entire flock. Or perhaps I catch sight of a murmuration of starlings, swarming in synchrony above my head. This pattern is a manifestation of a complex system in nature. Their synchronization serves to conserve energy and to protect individual birds who would otherwise be extremely vulnerable in the natural world.

Humans are animals too (at least for now), and we also have the capacity to communicate and synchronize in a rhythmic way. The small ways we witness this—a jazz quartet riffing in a nightclub, those amazing synchronized swimmers in the Olympics, or a sports team that seems undefeatable—manifest normative dissociation.

Entrainment and attunement are physical attributes of a complex system, and the subjective translation is a felt sense. It is easy to see the way in which entrainment facilitates survival in the flock of geese, or a murmuration of starlings. It is more difficult to fully appreciate it in the digitalized environment of modern, Westernized society (the population responsible for fossil fuel pollution and deforestation). With the loss of Indigenous scientific literacy, we have some leaders who not only fail to understand the natural forces of complex systems but do not recognize the survival value of empathy/attunement. Many bird species are capable of complex cognitive function, yet the lone goose in the sky is not "thinking" that if it flies in formation, it will conserve energy, or the lone starling is not "thinking" how to protect itself from a predator. They enter their formations automatically. And while many other species demonstrate some form of consciousness, human awareness is intertwined with complicated psychological phenomena. In the face of natural disasters, we often see an immediate human response of compassion and community collaboration. When faced with crises that require insight and planning, we are also seeing the emergence of other responses, tinged with greed and paranoia, raising the question, Can human psychology actually interfere with survival?

These questions envelop us in the psychotherapeutic process. What is the role of an analyst or therapist in helping individuals live in *this emerging* world? Clearly, we work to alleviate painful conflict and shame and self-injury with as much objectivity as possible—without cultural bias and with tolerance for difference. But if environmental changes threaten to destroy the possibility of well-being for our children and grandchildren, then do psychotherapists also have a mandate to recognize this institutional abuse, just as we are mandated to recognize individual abuse? Dobrich takes this further in her perspective about creating facilitative environments. She states,

> In communal life, this means nurturing spaces where people might feel held in their wholeness—where emotional awareness and attuned responsiveness can begin to emerge, even if imperfectly, offering an alternative to environments marked by judgment, dissociation, and neglect. Facilitative environments would also bear witness to the absence of these conditions, allowing what has been foreclosed to be acknowledged, thereby bringing the potential for connection, recognition, and transformation back online.
>
> (2026)

If we choose to look, we can see examples of individuals and organizations "bringing the potential for connection, recognition, and transformation back online." Since 2012,

> The Common Threads Project model, rooted in neuroscientific and sociocultural understanding of trauma, revives an ancient practice found in diverse contexts: women come together to sew their stories onto cloth, to disclose the *unspeakable* atrocities they have experienced, and to support one another. Common Threads Project integrates this tradition with best practices from trauma-informed therapy, bodywork, and psychoeducation.
>
> (Common Threads Project, n.d.)

In 2015 rural Scotland, a small group of people started a Climate Café, a place for some to talk about climate change concerns and for some to plan actions relevant to climate change concerns. Climate Cafés now exist on almost every continent on the globe and on the internet. From their website:

> The Climate Cafés® featured here all work to the same ethos—free, open, welcoming to all, inclusive, informal and a space to talk, listen, share and inspire action—without judgement or party politics or requiring particular expertise. They are often very creative spaces and benefit from intergenerational conversations.
>
> (Climate Café, n.d.)

Entrainment and attunement in our fragmented, digitalized society however, are not just about fostering embodied connection and community. We need to think about our emerging attunement to cyberlife, as well as human life. What does that actually mean? The recent short film *I Am Not a Robot*, directed by Victoria Warmerdam (2023), is a chilling representation of potential human-cyber attunement. Anyone treating children and adolescents knows there are ever-growing "communities" of gamers online, and many adults spend increasing amounts of time in a cyberworld. Can we make a connection between the flourishing of avatars and addictions to social media with an increasing tendency to just not think (know) about disturbing facts, like rising sea level, melting polar ice, and extreme weather events?

Just as we breathe pollutants in the air whether we know it or not, the concept of eco-neglect as child neglect informs our clinical work even if we never discuss it in a session. It is simply about noticing.

***

Noticing is a kind of waking up. I remember many moments of waking up, little "ahas" that had not been fully present in consciousness. As a young musician listening to Beethoven, I had the sudden awareness that without the silence in between the notes, there would be no shape to the music. As an older musician trying to learn something new (polyrhythmic drumming), I noticed that when I finally let go of my Western trained approach to playing music, then, like a miracle, my fingers would move in sync with the group, despite my having no clue in the moment how that was happening.

I often tell the story of trying to take my dog for a walk an hour before a thunderstorm. She does not make it very far down the path before she starts to tremble and refuses to move. She senses the oncoming storm before I have a clue about it. Her embodied awareness is never overruled by psychological defenses, and I can never force her to walk on.

Human beings, on the other hand, have evolved a tremendous capacity to override body awareness. This capacity is influenced by both an ability to deny and an ability to dissociate. Dissociation and denial can be intertwined. When we focus only on denial of the dangers of climate change, we are missing an opportunity to speak with vast numbers of individuals who are not in denial, but who are simply not paying attention—not looking and not listening and thereby experiencing variations of disconnected self-states. This reminds me of Katharine Hayhoe's concept of "psychological distance": that if it is not happening to me now, I am not noticing it (Hayhoe, 2021). Except that in actuality, it is happening to us now, and we are still not noticing it.

Let's go back to the first awareness of our pale blue dot for another example of the human capacity to notice and not know. On December 24, 1968, astronaut Bill Anders spontaneously took a photo of Earth during the Apollo 8 mission. The photo, later named *Earth Rise*, was unplanned. Of course, they knew that they were orbiting the earth. But they did not imagine what it would look like, and they did not realize that they would want to take the photo until the moment our planet appeared through the window of the spacecraft. I am listening to a recording of their voices as they scrambled to get the color film into the handheld camera. Anders can be heard saying, "Oh my God, look at that picture over there! There's the Earth comin' up. Wow, is that pretty!" (2018). These astronauts did not imagine, ahead of the mission, what Earth would look like from outer space and that they would feel an urgent need to take a photo.

There are many reasons why intelligent, capable human beings both don't pay attention and sometimes fail to imagine. And of course, there are exceptions to that failure. In 1993, the Afrofuturist writer Octavia Butler wrote the novel *Parable of the Sower*, in which she so presciently imagined the devastating impact of climate changes and social inequities in the year 2024.

Twenty-two years after the Apollo 8 mission, in 1990, a photo of Earth taken by Voyager I as it was leaving our solar system was named the *Pale Blue Dot* by astronomer Carl Sagan. Sagan had a keen awareness of strife and petty struggles among human inhabitants of Earth. He wrote, "Our posturings, our imagined self-importance, the delusion that we have some privileged position in the Universe, are challenged by this point of pale light" (1994, p. 7). These days, as human evolution is catapulting toward an intersection with artificial intelligence, scientists and philosophers like David Chalmers (2022) are asking the question, Are we living in a simulation? When I am sitting in my quiet, little office, face-to-face, in person or online, such a question feels entirely irrelevant. And the "delusion" of a privileged position in the universe feels potentially tragic. Psychotherapists and psychoanalysts sit at the intersection of individual and social consciousness, often with way too much information to make sense of what we are noticing. What we do with individuals and/or small groups can be the equivalent of spontaneously snapping that photo of Earth. Simply helping humans to look, listen, and to notice.

References

Anders, Bill. (2018, December 21). The story behind Apollo 8's famous earthrise photo. *NASA*. https://science.nasa.gov/resource/the-story-behind-apollo-8s-famous-earthrise-photo/

Apprey, M. (2023). *Transgenerational haunting in psychoanalysis*. Routledge.

Bourdillon, M., Driscoll J. J., Myers, W., O'Kane, C., & Rink, P. (2024). Climate crisis as a form of structural violence against children and youth. *BMJ Paediatrics Open*, *8*(1), 1.

Bromberg, P. (1999). *Standing in the spaces: Essays on clinical process, trauma, and dissociation*. Routledge.

Bucci, W. (2021). *Emotional communication and therapeutic change: Understanding psychotherapy through multiple code theory* (W. F. Cornell, Ed.). Routledge.

Butler, O. E. (1993). *Parable of the sower*. Four Walls Eight Windows.

Butler, L. D. (2006). Normative dissociation. *The Psychiatric Clinics of North America*, *29*(1), 45–62.

Chalmers, D. J. (2022). *Reality +: Virtual worlds and the problems of philosophy*. Norton.

Chefetz, R. (2015). *Intensive psychotherapy for persistent dissociative processes: The fear of feeling real*. Norton.

Committee on the Rights of the Child. (2023). General comment No. 26 (2023) on children's rights and the environment with a special focus on climate change (CRC/C/GC/26). United Nations. https://www.ohchr.org/en/documents/general-comments-and-recommendations/crccgc26-general-comment-no-26-2023-childrens-rights

Common Threads Project. (n.d.). https://commonthreadsproject.org/

Dobrich, J. (2021). *Working with survivor siblings in psychoanalysis: Ability and disability in clinical process* (1st ed.). Routledge.

Dobrich, J. (2026). Conclusion: The "field" as patient: Psychoanalytic practice beyond the individual. In J. Dobrich (Ed.), *Moving from grievance to hope in psychoanalysis: Applied case studies*. (pp. 217–225). Routledge.

Gendlin, E. T. (1981). *Focusing*. Bantam

Hayhoe, K. (2021). *Saving us: A climate scientist's case for hope and healing in a divided world.* Simon & Schuster.

Hopenwasser K. (2008). Being in rhythm: Dissociative attunement in therapeutic process. *Journal of Trauma & Dissociation*, *9*(3):349–367. https://doi.org/10.1080/15299730802139212

Hopenwasser, K. (2016). Dissociative attunement in a resonant world. In L. Howell & S. Izkowitz (Eds.), *The dissociative mind in psychoanalysis* (pp. 175–186). Routledge.

Hopenwasser K. (2024). Understanding the role of trauma and dissociation in youth responses to climate crises: Eco-neglect as institutional child abuse. In E. Haase & K. Hudson (Eds.), *Climate change and youth mental health: Multidisciplinary perspectives* (pp. 130–147). Cambridge University Press.

Howell, E., & Itzkowitz, S. (Eds.). (2016). *The dissociative mind in psychoanalysis: Understanding and working with trauma* (1st ed.). Routledge.

Kempe, C. H., Silverman, F. N., Steele, B. F., Droegemuerller, W., & Silver, H. K. (1962). The battered-child syndrome. *Journal of the American Medical Association*, *181*(1), 17–24.

Knoblauch, S. (2020). *Bodies and social rhythms: Navigating unconscious vulnerability and emotional fluidity* (1st ed.). Routledge.

Laub, D., & Auerhahn, N. C. (1993). Knowing and not knowing massive psychic trauma: Forms of traumatic memory. *The International Journal of Psycho-Analysis*, *74*(2), 287–302.

Mucci, C. (2013). *Beyond individual and collective trauma: Intergenerational transmission, psychoanalytic treatment, and the dynamics of forgiveness* (1st ed.). Routledge.

Mucci, C. (2022). *Resilience and survival: Understanding and healing intergenerational trauma*. Confer Books.

Orange, D. M. (2017). *Climate crisis, psychoanalysis, and radical ethics*. Routledge.

Orange, D. M. (2020). *Psychoanalysis, history, and radical ethics: Learning to hear*. Routledge.

Our Children's Trust. (n.d.). https://www.ourchildrenstrust.org

Sagan, C. (1980). *Cosmos: A personal voyage*. Random House.

Sagan, C. (1994). *Pale blue dot: A vision of the human future in space*. Random House.

Saidipour, P. (2020). The precedent of good enough therapy during unprecedented times. *Clnical Social Work Journal*, *49*(4), 429–436.

Salberg, J., & Grand, S. (2016). *Wounds of history: Repair and resilience in the transgenerational transmission of trauma*. Routledge.

Solnit, R. (2018). Climate change is violence. In R. Solnit (Ed.), *Call them by their true names: American crises (and essays)* (pp. 83–87). Haymarket Books.

Stern, D. B. (2003). *Unformulated experience: From dissociation to imagination in psychoanalysis* (1st ed.). Routledge.

The Climate Café. (n.d.). About. https://www.climate.cafe/about/

Tosone, C., Nuttman-Shwartz, O., & Stephens, T. (2012). Shared trauma: When the professional is personal. *Clinical Social Work Journal*, *40*, 231–239.

Trevarthen, C. (1999–2000). Musicality and the intrinsic motive pulse: Evidence from human psychobiology and infant communication. *Musicae Scientiae, Special Issue*, 155–215.

United Nations Committee on the Rights of the Child. (2023). Report of the Committee on the Rights of the Child, 90th session (3 May–3 June 2022), 91st session (29 August–23 September 2022), 92nd session (16 January–3 February 2023), 93rd session (8–26 May 2023), 94th session (4–22 September 2023), 95th session (15 January–2 February 2024). United Nations. https://digitallibrary.un.org/record/4059139

Volkan, V. D. (2001). Transgenerational transmissions and chosen traumas: An aspect of large-group identity. *Group Analysis*, *34*(1), 79–97. https://doi.org/10.1177/05333160122077730

Walsh, Z., Böhme, J., & Wamsler, C. (2021). Towards a relational paradigm in sustainability research, practice, and education. *Ambio*, *50*(1), 74–84.

Warmerdam, V. (Director). (2023). *I'm not a robot* [Short film]. *The New Yorker*.

Weintrobe, S. (2021). *Psychological roots of climate consciousness: Neoliberal exceptionalism and the culture of uncare*. Bloomsbury Academic.

West, S., Haider, L. J., Hertz, T., Mancilla Garcia, M., & Moore, M. L. (2024). Relational approaches to sustainability transformations: Walking together in a world of many worlds. *Ecosystems and People*, *20*(1). https://doi.org/10.1080/26395916.2024.2370539

West, S., Haider, L. J., Stålhammar, S., & Woroniecki, S. (2020). A relational turn for sustainability science? Relational thinking, leverage points and transformations. *Ecosystems and People*, *16*(1), 304–325. https://doi.org/10.1080/26395916.2020.1814417

Conclusion

The "Field" as Patient: Psychoanalytic Practice Beyond the Individual

Johanna Dobrich

The collection of essays in this volume each illuminates distinct psychoanalytic contributions to nurturing pluralistic generativity in communal life, both within specific subgroups and in the connections between diverse communities. By *facing* what remains unformulated and/or aggrieved within the self, the community, and the wider field, psychoanalytic resonance engages the field itself, guiding it back toward potential space and away from the polarization born of fusion and concreteness[1] (Winnicott, 1971). By *facing*, I do not mean a singular or linear act of recognition but rather an ongoing relational capacity to hold the ambiguity, contradiction, and emotional tension within pain without retreating fully into defensiveness or dissociation—to remain present and listening in the face of dialectical tensions that cannot be easily resolved or integrated into full understanding but must coexist. A facilitative environment resists the urge to erase, minimize, or simplify painful or unresolved circumstances and clashes. It halts any action in the service of first formulating and understanding. Instead, it sustains communal attunement to what is difficult, unknown, or incomplete, while witnessing what hurts. Such environments draw on psychoanalytic concepts of mentalization particularly of dissociative experience (Fonagy et al., 2002), the capacity to hold paradox (Winnicott, 1965/1971), and the ethic of witnessing (Benjamin, 2018; Orange, 2020). Together, these frameworks deepen our ability to remain present to complexity within ourselves and others, as well as across the broader social field.

Winnicott's notion of the facilitative environment is especially apropos in applied psychoanalysis, which is not outcome-driven but instead attends to atmosphere—creating, sustaining, and maintaining a place in which individual and communal maturation and development can

DOI: 10.4324/9781003658382-11

go on being (Winnicott, 1965). Just as an infant relies on a good-enough caregiver to create a facilitative environment that nurtures the emergence of an authentic, cohesive self, *sovereign communities* rest upon supportive atmospheres that allow individuals and groups to develop authentic relationships and intersubjective relationality with one another. In communal life, this means maintaining spaces where people might feel held in their wholeness, where self/emotional awareness and attuned responsiveness can begin to emerge, even if imperfectly, offering an alternative to environments marked by judgment, destruction, dissociation, hierarchal posturing, and neglect. Facilitative environments also bear witness to the absence of these conditions when they are inevitably threatened or interrupted, allowing what has been foreclosed to be acknowledged, thereby bringing the potential for connection, recognition, and transformation back online.

Pathology in the social field consistently reveals a collapse or foreclosure of potential space, the vital intermediate area where imagination, symbolization, and emotional processing occur (Winnicott, 1971). When this space is compromised, communities become trapped in rigid, defensive states marked by dissociation and/or grievance, which belie an inability to mourn and transition. Without the holding and containing function of potential space, communities struggle to transform traumatic experiences into post-traumatic resiliency, perpetuating cycles of despair, violence, and further fragmentation. Restoring this space is essential for enabling collective healing, expansion, and emergence of new possibilities within the social psyche. As psychoanalysts, we are trained to listen deeply to the echoes of cultural life within the individual psyche, attuned to how desire, despair, potential, and destruction coexist and collide. This nuanced listening allows us to perceive the complex interplay between personal and collective experience, revealing the often-hidden tensions that shape both inner worlds and social realities. Not everyone has this kind of capacity developed, and those who do have a vital role to play.

A facilitative environment at the communal level ultimately fosters epistemic trust, an awareness of our interdependency, mutual care, and a commitment to finding shared meaning-making, creating a space where individuals can experience their vulnerabilities without fear of absolute fragmentation, annihilation, or rejection. Fonagy et al. (2015) notion of epistemic trust refers to a capacity to trust the information communicated by others as relevant, reliable, and personally meaningful. This trust is what opens the door for learning and change, especially in relational contexts. When epistemic trust is established, individuals become receptive to new knowledge and can revise maladaptive beliefs or patterns as well as engage across difference. Conversely, disruptions in epistemic trust, often rooted in early relational trauma at both the individual and social level, can lead to defensive withdrawal, skepticism, and social disengagement, limiting the possibility for understanding, growth, and connection.

In other words, facilitative environments provide the "holding" function at a collective level, naming, containing, and translating anxiety, fear,[2] anger, and tension to help groups navigate conflict and difference *constructively* (Winnicott, 1965). For example, Volkan (2004) positions the psychoanalyst as a reflective "third" one who listens for the unspoken, and helps surface collective trauma and identity wounds, creating space for mourning and meaning-making, so that groups loosen rigid narratives and begin to *imagine* one another differently. Without psychoanalysts serving as anchors to create such an environment, communities risk becoming fragmented or defensive, leading to ideological adaptations, such as conformity, suppression of dissent, violent "solutions," and the scapegoating of self/others, that may protect against relational threat but inhibit intersubjective connection and growth (Berger, 2018). As ideology replaces relationality, societies' intrapsychic, interpersonal, and collective struggles become entrenched and inhibited. Absent any agents available to promote Winnicott's facilitative environment, groups fixate and marinate in grievance and conflicts ossify. Applied psychoanalysis highlights the role educator-clinicians may play in nurturing psychological and relational health from within families to neighborhoods, organizations, and wider social systems, alongside other actors such as religious figures, nonprofit leaders, and humanistic visionaries. When communal environments are facilitative, they support the ongoing development of both individual and collective capacities for resilience, creativity, maturation, and belonging.

The clinician-educators in this series demonstrate how this work can take shape through active listening and resonance—both outward and inward—through the facilitation and formulating of lived experiences, tolerating paradox and complexity without rushing or attempting to resolve it, and, perhaps most essentially, through recognizing that the human condition is marked by grieving what has been lost in order to make space for what is yet to come. Accompanying one another in that ongoing process brings us back to our roots as psychoanalysts. Nurturing communities in their capacity to witness provides the vital platform where these tasks can be addressed collectively, something policymakers, ideologically driven leaders, and unattuned systems are not equipped to offer. As psychoanalysts, we hold a unique place in carrying forward Freud's profound realization that mourning is necessary alchemy, and we are uniquely equipped to bear witness to this at the communal level, providing the space and support necessary for its unfolding (1917). Mourning invites us to face loss and grief without rushing toward any premature resolution or denial, allowing the psyche the time and space to transform pain into deepened subjectivity and ultimately enlivened connection. In this work, we do not only witness loss; we also bear witness to growth, transformation, and the gains that emerge through struggle. In community contexts, this dual witnessing of both losses and gains becomes essential, as collective experiences of trauma and resilience coexist, demanding reflection and containment to foster integration and growth. Tangible support and changes in the social structure and policy are absolutely components of change, but without a facilitative environment, these practices alone often fall short of creating the desired outcome of *vitalizing* communal life that remains at the heart of the psychoanalytic enterprise. Psychoanalysts such as Eigen (1993), Schwartz-Cooney and Sopher (2020), and Ogden (2019) have emphasized the importance of awakening vitalization through the psychoanalytic process, the reawakening or sustaining of life's creative and emotional energy within the individual. This process goes beyond mere symptom relief to engage the living, dynamic aspects of the psyche, facilitating a deeper connection with one's vitality and aliveness.

I perceive a common thread woven through each of these chapters, a thread that illuminates how psychoanalysts help create or sustain witnessing communities: a sacred space where the clash of inner and relational struggles can be seen, held gently, understood deeply, and, at times, transformed. When actors driven primarily by ego and self-interest, as opposed to collective good, are in positions of leadership, sometimes all we can offer is working toward the maintenance and sustenance of witnessing communities and the preservation of some potential space to call in less polarizing and fragmented leadership and psychologically stuck citizenry. For example, Shapiro (2005, 2020), drawing from systems-centered and psychoanalytic perspectives, views leadership as a relational and systemic function that goes beyond the individual. He emphasizes that leaders carry the projections and anxieties of the group, becoming a container for unspoken tensions, conflicts, or desires, a tall task to manage. If they are focused primarily on exercising their authority, the capacity to transform and to lead is deeply impaired. Shapiro presents a psychoanalytic framework for effective leadership, emphasizing the delicate balancing of boundaries, the facilitation of reflective space, and the vital role leaders play in helping groups bear complexity and ambiguity, particularly when under pressure. Ultimately, leadership is less about authority and more about *helping systems think about themselves*. By humanizing those we oppose, bearing witness to their legitimate grievances, and resisting the impulse to reduce them to caricatures of Other, we create a vital space for mourning, containment, and its aftermath. It is within this holding environment that dialogue, relationality, and difference can coexist: crucial elements in the psychic alchemy that transforms grievance into possibility.

Just like the early environment of the family life, social life occurs within a communal environment with profound impact on what we can come to express and know. The social field can either lean toward supporting or constraining the process of healthy relationality and intersubjective knowing. In the context of community psychoanalysis, each contributor employs tools and methods that help bring unconscious group dynamics into view, particularly phenomena such as projective identification, splitting, forestalled mourning, and traumatic reenactments, which unfold across social and institutional terrains wrecking damage and engendering a nonfacilitative reactive cycle. The dynamics rooted in individual psyches become amplified in community settings, where histories of trauma, marginalization, and power asymmetries live on in potent ways. Through careful observation, deep listening, skilled facilitation capacities, and reflective engagement, psychoanalysis has a role to play in decoding the communications that occur at the group level. Navigating transference and countertransference in these contexts requires an ongoing attunement to how our internal worlds intersect with collective experience. By staying with these tensions without taking sides, we begin to illuminate the unconscious forces shaping our social worlds and open *the possibility* for more generative forms of connection and repair. In the absence of facilitative environments and system-wise leadership, the witnessing that community psychoanalysis nurtures become all the more critical.

Across the varied clinical terrains explored in this volume, creating potential space through the development of witnessing communities involves reaching beyond the traditional edges of care, placing psychoanalytic work within a wider fabric of social attunement, ethical response, and collective possibility (Hopenwasser, 2026). This expanded framework navigates the interplay between inner psychic realities and the external conditions of displacement, disaster, oppression, and marginalization (Wyatt & Beznes, 2026). Recognizing the archetypal dimensions of these issues is crucial to understanding their depth and their resistance to simple solutions (Fromm, 2026; Gross Nathenson, 2026). Central to this work is a willingness to confront either shadow material or it's contemporary cousins unformulated or disavowed experience—both individual and collective (Frie, 2026; Sidesinger, 2026). Without such confrontation, cycles of moral reactivity persist, obstructing the capacity to metabolize the complex emotions and disavowed experiences that underlie conflict (Fromm, 2026; Gross Nathenson, 2026). Boulanger (2007) sees the integration of aggression as central to recovery from war and catastrophic man-made trauma. Survivors must come to know not only what was done to them but also who they had to become in order to survive, including their aggressive capacities, and to hold that knowledge without psychic collapse (Grand, 2000). Embracing social responsibility requires the difficult but necessary task of shadow integration: cultivating reflection on our own contradictions, aggression, and complexity without reflexively locating them in the "other side" (Gross Nathenson, 2026). Through attuned resonance, the engagement of processes that foster self-reclamation, and a focus on attachment dynamics within marginal and intersectional identities, psychoanalysts may support the emergence of sovereignty alongside affiliation, as well as the possibility of post-traumatic growth (Dobrich, 2026; Fromm, 2026; Pivnick, 2026). Multimodal, culturally responsive psychoanalytic care has been especially vital in communities impacted by trauma and dislocation, meeting communities in the fullness of what they need, beyond the confines of the consulting room (Cerfolio, 2026; Wyatt & Beznes, 2026).

Collaborative consultation with community stakeholders emphasizes the analyst's role in holding and witnessing the process, supporting rather than directing, and trusting the group's own capacity to discover solutions together. This stance embodies a profound respect for the unfolding work of transformation. Engagement with multiple modalities such as art-making, pottery, writing, and reflective workshops, enriches the container, inviting alternative ways of knowing and expression into community building. Ultimately, these efforts reflect a commitment to careful observation, to remaining present with what emerges, and to containing the complexity, contradiction, and potential within the social field. Facilitating containment, securing a place from which to "see," and promoting intersubjective dialogue are core practices that support the process of symbolization and ultimately intersubjective life. It is through these relational and reflective acts that we begin to represent our inner and outer experiences. Once we are able to symbolize rather than only enact and react, a space opens for integration, meaning-making, and the possibility of creative living.

Psychoanalysts may serve as cross-cultural translators, helping communities learn how to hear themselves more deeply and to discover more agentic ways of being recognized and met. In this way, symbolization becomes both a psychological *and* communal achievement, rooted in the capacity to hold and reflect upon experience together. Psychoanalysts can help turn a static environment into a facilitative one by listening to narratives not as fixed, factual accounts, but as *poems*: as expressions layered with rhythm, tone, and metaphor. In doing so, we invite meaning to emerge not through linear logic, but through resonance. Metaphor becomes a crucial tool here: a way to carry and communicate experience across divides that might otherwise feel insurmountable. We also learn to attune to the wounded demand for recognition, not as resistance or pathology, but as an expression of hidden or obscured loss, which, when held and acknowledged, allows patterns of entitlement to soften. Before engaging in debate at the cognitive level, psychoanalysis may first help communities return to their *bodies*, to find grounding and presence in sensation and emotion, enlisting imagination—not as an escape, but as one of the most powerful capacities we have to soften the defensive system, reanimate inner life, and create the conditions for something new to unfold.

Notes

1 *Cancel culture* and *assassination culture* exemplify what occurs when the social *field* becomes rigidly entrenched in grievance, with opposing sides seeing the "solution" as the annihilation of the Other. Moral injury, regardless of its severity, demands accountability and then mourning—not destruction of the Other—for renewal to arise (Herman, 2023).

2 The evocative title of *We Don't Speak of Fear: Large-Group Identity, Societal Conflict and Collective Trauma* captures the critical importance of naming fear in particular, as the collective fears that go unspoken yet shape large-group identity and intergroup conflict remain a prominent affect (Volkan, Scholz, & Fromm, 2023).

References

Benjamin, J. (2018). *Beyond doer and done to: Recognition theory, intersubjectivity and the third*. Routledge.

Berger, J. M. (2018). *Extremism*. Massachusetts Institute of Technology Press.

Boulanger, G. (2007). *Wounded by reality: Understanding and treating adult-onset trauma*. Analytic Press.

Cerfolio, N. (2026). From destruction to growth: Multimodal psychoanalytic aid for war-traumatized Chechen children. In J. Dobrich (Ed.), *Moving from grievance to hope in psychoanalysis: Applied case studies*. (pp. 39–58). Routledge.

Dobrich, J. (2026). Ethnocultural identity and attachment: Unraveling legacies of self-erasure. In J. Dobrich (Ed.), *Moving from grievance to hope in psychoanalysis: Applied case studies*. (pp. 170–204). Routledge.

Eigen, M. (1993). *Vitalization in psychoanalysis*. Routledge.

Fonagy, P., Gergely, G., Jurist, E. L., & Target, M. (2002). *Affect regulation, mentalization, and the development of the self*. Other Press.

Fonagy, P., Luyten, P., & Allison, E. (2015). Epistemic petrification and the restoration of epistemic trust: A new conceptualization of borderline personality disorder and its psychosocial treatment. *Journal of Personality Disorders*, *29*(5), 575–609. https://doi.org/10.1521/pedi.2015.29.5.575

Freud, S. (1917). Mourning and melancholia. In J. Strachey (Ed. & Trans.), *The standard edition of the complete psychological works of Sigmund Freud* (Vol. 14, pp. 237–258). Hogarth Press. (Original work published 1915).

Frie, R. (2026). Social psychoanalysis, silencing, and racial violence. In J. Dobrich (Ed.), *Moving from grievance to hope in psychoanalysis: Applied case studies*. (pp. 59–78). Routledge.

Fromm, M. G. (2026). Traveling through time: A group intervention in Northern Ireland. In J. Dobrich (Ed.), *Moving from grievance to hope in psychoanalysis: Applied case studies*. (pp. 79–95). Routledge.

Grand, S. (2000). *The reproduction of evil: A clinical and cultural perspective*. Analytic Press.

Gross Nathenson, R. (2026). A Jungian perspective on mass shootings, American gun culture, and psychoanalysis. In J. Dobrich (Ed.), *Moving from grievance to hope in psychoanalysis: Applied case studies*. (pp. 113–134). Routledge.

Herman, J. L. (2023). *Trauma and recovery: The aftermath of violence—From domestic abuse to political terror* (2nd ed.). Basic Books.

Hopenwasser, K. (2026). Knowing and not knowing about our climate crisis: From eco-neglect to mutual sustenance on planet Earth. In J. Dobrich (Ed.), *Moving from grievance to hope in psychoanalysis: Applied case studies*. (pp. 205–216). Routledge.

Ogden, T. H. (2019). *What "alive" means: Psychoanalytic explorations of subjectivity, theory, and being human*. Routledge.

Orange, D. M. (2020). *Psychoanalysis, history, and radical ethics: Learning to hear*. Routledge.

Pivnick, B. (2026). Grievance, grief, and group building in community psychoanalysis. In J. Dobrich (Ed.), *Moving from grievance to hope in psychoanalysis: Applied case studies*. (pp. 135–169). Routledge.

Schwartz-Cooney, L., & Sopher, D. (Eds.). (2020). *Vitalization in psychoanalysis: Perspectives on being and becoming*. Routledge.

Shapiro, E. R. (2005). The inner world in the outer world: Psychoanalytic concepts in organizational settings. In L. S. Rafael & V. L. Green (Eds.), *Group dynamics and organizational culture: Effective work groups and organizations* (pp. 99–113). SAGE Publications.

Shapiro, E. R. (2020). *Finding a place to stand: Developing self-reflective institutions, leaders and citizens*. Phoenix Publishing House.

Sidesinger, T. (2026). Writing matrescence: Therapeutic writing retreats as collective containers for transgenerational healing. In J. Dobrich (Ed.), *Moving from grievance to hope in psychoanalysis: Applied case studies*. (pp. 96–112). Routledge.

Volkan, V. D. (2004). *Blind trust: Large groups and their leaders in times of crisis and terror*. Pitchstone Publishing.

Volkan, V. D., Scholz, R., & Fromm, M. G. (Eds.). (2023). *We don't speak of fear: Large-group identity, societal conflict and collective trauma*. Phoenix Publishing House.

Winnicott, D. W. (1965). *The maturational processes and the facilitating environment: Studies in the theory of emotional development*. International Universities Press.

Winnicott, D. W. (1971). *Playing and reality*. Tavistock Publications.

Wyatt, R., & Beznes, A. (2026). Beyond borders: Psychoanalytic perspectives on refugee healing. In J. Dobrich (Ed.), *Moving from grievance to hope in psychoanalysis: Applied case studies*. Routledge.

Index

Please note that page numbers in **bold** denote tables, while n indicates an endnote.

For Product Safety Concerns and Information please contact our EU representative GPSR@taylorandfrancis.com
Taylor & Francis Verlag GmbH, Kaufingerstraße 24, 80331 München, Germany

www.ingramcontent.com/pod-product-compliance
Lightning Source LLC
Chambersburg PA
CBHW070244230726
48635CB00031B/424
9781041110408